# Alzheimer's
# Through the Stages

*A Caregiver's Guide*

# Alzheimer's Through the Stages

*A Caregiver's Guide*

What to Expect, What to Say,
What to Do

Mary Moller, MSW, CAS

ALTHEA
PRESS

For general information on our other products and services or to obtain technical support, please contact our Customer Care Department within the United States at (866) 744-2665, or outside the United States at (510) 253-0500.

Althea Press publishes its books in a variety of electronic and print formats. Some content that appears in print may not be available in electronic books, and vice versa.

Interior and Cover Designer: Joshua Moore
Photo Art Director: Sara Feinstein
Editor: Melissa Valentine
Production Editor: Andrew Yackira

ISBN: Print 978-1-64152-270-0 | eBook 978-1-64152-271-7

To Randy, Wyatt, Luke,
Bebe, and Pop

# Contents

# Introduction

" There are only four kinds of people: those who will become caregivers, those who are caregivers, those who were caregivers, and those who'll need caregiving themselves." —ROSALYNN CARTER

For you, becoming a caregiver may have been expected, unexpected, by choice, or by chance. Regardless of your reason for becoming a caregiver, this part of the caregiving journey has brought you to this book.

You probably have questions. You may wonder, what does the future hold? How can I possibly help? You may feel alone. I promise, you are not. You are embarking on a journey with millions of others who are caring right now for the estimated 5.7 million people with Alzheimer's in America today.

By the time you're reaching out for this information, your loved one may be well past the early stages of Alzheimer's disease. The changes in your loved one may have been going on for several years. In retrospect, you may look back and realize that the warning signs were all there. Now, that being said, be reassured that it's very common for those who are closest to their loved ones to not fully realize what's happening. During the early stages, the older adult may be able to explain away forgetfulness, misplacing things, fender benders, not paying bills or double paying bills, and so forth. In fact, most people believe that changes in memory, thinking, or behavior are a normal part of aging and growing old. To some degree, they can be; however, sometimes these can be signs that something bigger is happening.

Don't be hard on yourself—none of us know what the future holds, and we certainly don't expect Alzheimer's disease to be part of it. Looking back and recognizing that this may have been developing over time is a normal reaction. Alzheimer's disease is a progressive neuro-degenerative disease that takes many years to progress and evolve.

For over 15 years, I've had the privilege of working with caregivers in a variety of capacities. Initially, I was hired to develop a new and innovative program that would provide support services to caregivers. One of the first caregivers I met said to me, "When I took my wedding vows and said, 'For better or worse; in sickness and in health,' no one told me about Alzheimer's disease." I'll never forget her, a lovely lady married for over 40 years, suddenly charged with taking care of her husband. From that moment on, I knew that caregivers were special people and unsung heroes.

As the program evolved, I facilitated hundreds of caregiver support groups and coordinated a variety of support services for older adults with cognitive impairment and their caregivers. In working with caregivers, it quickly became clear that many caregivers put their own needs aside and focus all their time and energy on caring for their loved ones. This leads countless caregivers to compromise their own health and wellness, especially as the older adults with memory loss increasingly rely on them. As the needs and dependencies of the older adults become more comprehensive, the caregivers have less time and energy to take care of themselves. This realization has led me to identify caregiver health and wellness as an important priority for caregivers. From the first doctor's appointment onward, caregivers must take care of themselves.

I currently work at the Center of Excellence for Alzheimer's Disease at Albany Medical Center in New York, surrounded by a team of caring, compassionate healthcare experts. This experience has reaffirmed my commitment to promoting the health and wellness of the caregiver, and at the core of this journey, the older adult with Alzheimer's disease. My colleagues exemplify how to treat people with dignity and respect in all stages of the disease, and I'm pleased to share what I've learned from them so you can do the same.

When a loved one with Alzheimer's disease is unaware of or unclear about their surroundings, and they may not recognize who is helping them and why, compassion and kindness are truly humanitarian efforts given from the heart. You, as a caregiver, may never be thanked; your loved one may forget you the moment you leave the room, especially in the later stages of the disease. This commitment is not about accolades, nor even the satisfaction of helping them recover—it's about providing the best care possible when a loved one is in their greatest time of need.

In recent years, I've had a tremendous opportunity to specialize in Alzheimer's disease and dementia training and education. As part of this, I'm able to focus on the crucial issues of caregiver health and wellness. Through educational workshops, trainings, and presentations, I address topics such as compassion fatigue, caregiver stress, and burnout. The more I've been able to interact with these unsung heroes, the more passionate I've become. Caregiver health and wellness and self-care have become professional and personal priorities for me!

Indeed, skilled and compassionate healthcare providers are so very integral to the continuum of care. But I've come to recognize that at the center of it all stands the caregiver, who remains the most important part of the care plan, from the diagnosis onward.

For the past 15 years, I've been saying, "When caregivers take care of themselves, they are better able to care for their loved ones." It's so true. Those who care for an older adult with Alzheimer's disease are at increased risk for depression, higher levels of stress, and caregiver burnout. Caregiver isolation also tends to increase as the disease progresses through the stages. As the level and complexity of care increases, the burden on the caregiver can become all-consuming.

I am delighted to provide this book as a guide to help make sure you are equipped with the information, guidance, and support you'll need along this journey. I want to help you be the best caregiver you can be, to both yourself and your loved one.

Many caregivers compare this part of their lives to a roller-coaster ride—lots of ups and downs with twists and turns, dark tunnels, and bright passages. This book will help you navigate the next chapter in your life, as a caregiver for an older adult with Alzheimer's disease. In this book, you'll learn practical tips and strategies to help reduce caregiver stress, as well as real-world solutions to various issues. You'll hear stories that you may be able to relate to as a caregiver, and I'll offer some methods that can contribute to a successful daily routine and make transitions easier, if not more predictable. This book is meant to be used as an ongoing supportive resource as you encounter uncharted territory or a difficult situation as a caregiver. When you need accurate information, guidance, reassurance, support, motivation, and inspiration, this book is here for you.

Alzheimer's disease generally progresses slowly over time, and everyone experiences symptoms differently. My colleagues at our local Alzheimer's Association chapter often say, "When you've met one person with Alzheimer's disease, you've met one person with Alzheimer's disease." It's true! Even with 5.7 million people in America suffering from Alzheimer's, every one of those people and their caregivers experiences the disease differently. As a side note, you'll see references throughout this book to the Alzheimer's Association. This trusted resource and hub for international research is available for all of us to access for expert, accurate, and up-to-date information.

What we *do* know is that there are similarities across the stages of the disease that contribute to the neurodegenerative process. Several schools of thought describe the progression of Alzheimer's disease: According to the National Institutes of Health and the Alzheimer's Association, there are three general stages of the disease: mild, moderate, and severe. According to the National Institute on Aging, the disease progression is identified in terms of early, middle, and late stages.

Another more detailed method categorizes the progression of Alzheimer's disease in seven stages. These stages will also be described throughout the book. It can be helpful to learn these stages to better understand the disease progression:

> **Stage 1** – *No cognitive impairment*
>
> **Stage 2** – *Very mild cognitive decline*
>
> **Stage 3** – *Mild cognitive decline*
>
> **Stage 4** – *Moderate cognitive decline*
>
> **Stage 5** – *Moderate to severe cognitive decline*
>
> **Stage 6** – *Severe cognitive decline*
>
> **Stage 7** – *Very severe cognitive decline*

As every person experiences the disease differently, you'll notice that the definitions of the stages are somewhat fluid. There can be significant overlap between the stages; therefore, using the broader definitions interchangeably is common and acceptable—mild/early, moderate/middle, and severe/late. We'll refer to them all frequently in this book.

Between the terminology and the uncertainty of what lies ahead, your head may be spinning. The important thing to remember is that this book is full of information that will be available to support you, the caregiver, throughout the progression of the disease. You are not alone on this journey! However, it's true that no matter how much information you have at your fingertips, watching your loved one descend into a different reality can be extraordinarily difficult for the caregiver and everyone who is close to them. It can't be stated more clearly that, as a caregiver, you are your loved one's most important ally on this journey into the world of Alzheimer's disease. Be gentle with yourself, and know that you are so very special—the fact that you care enough to pick up this book demonstrates that you'll do the very best you can, given the circumstances that have been thrust upon you. As the Chinese philosopher Lao Tzu once stated, "From caring comes courage."

# PART ONE

# ALZHEIMER'S 101

We'll start with the basics, clarifying the differences between Alzheimer's disease and dementia. We'll also address the invaluable role that caregivers take on this journey called Alzheimer's disease.

CHAPTER ONE

# What Is Alzheimer's Disease?

I n this first chapter, we'll spend time learning about the basics of Alzheimer's disease and gathering some of the information that will help you navigate through the stages. You'll come to understand:

- the difference between Alzheimer's disease and dementia
- what you can expect in the different stages of Alzheimer's disease
- some common symptoms that people experience
- the important role of caregivers on this journey

## Dementia and Alzheimer's

Most people believe that Alzheimer's disease and dementia are two different diseases. In fact, Alzheimer's is a form of dementia. Dementia is a neurodegenerative disease that results in progressive and irreversible damage and loss of neurons that impair brain functioning.

"Dementia" broadly describes changes in the brain that cause difficulties with thinking, problem solving, judgment, and memory. Dementia also encompasses many symptoms, such as changes in behaviors, memory, thinking, reasoning, and managing emotions, along with a general loss of cognitive functioning. These symptoms progress over time, often taking years to develop and interfering more and more with daily life and routine activities. Every person with dementia experiences the process differently, and the time it takes for dementia to impact various parts of the brain is different for every person.

It's important to note that there are many types of dementia. Various disorders and factors contribute to the development of dementia.

These neurodegenerative diseases result in a progressive and irreversible loss of neurons and brain functioning, and currently, there is no cure.

## HOW ALZHEIMER'S WORKS

There are many types and causes of dementia, but Alzheimer's is the most common. Of all the diagnosed cases of dementia, as many as 60 to 80 percent are classified as Alzheimer's disease. Alzheimer's disease causes problems with memory, thinking, reasoning, and behaviors. Symptoms develop slowly over several years and get worse over time, eventually becoming severe enough to interfere with daily life, and ultimately all functioning abilities. Although there are things you can do to positively impact the trajectory (and we will discuss them in this book), there is currently no cure for Alzheimer's disease, and the damage that occurs over the years is irreversible. Alzheimer's disease destroys cells in the brain called neurons. Neurons are cells in the nervous system that transmit communication to each other—this communication directs and regulates all the actions in the human body, both voluntary and involuntary, that are necessary for survival.

Think of the brain as the control tower that sends information throughout the body—the neurons are the messengers. As Alzheimer's disease destroys and interrupts the communication between the neurons, this causes disruptions in memory, thinking, and other functions that require processing information.

Alzheimer's disease generally starts in the part of the brain called the hippocampus. The hippocampus is a critical part of the brain responsible for memory. The hippocampus also helps us with orientation, which is directly connected to memory. For example, the hippocampus tells us where we put our keys, how to use the washing machine, and how to make breakfast. All of the thinking that directs the functions and activities that we use all day, every day, is directed by the hippocampus. Alzheimer's disease slowly attacks the hippocampus by creating plaques and tangles—structures that kill neurons. The neurons die off because they can no longer communicate with each other and are starved of essential nutrients needed for life and functioning. Alzheimer's symptoms may begin with mild memory loss, possibly leading to an inability to remember names or events or to respond to changes in environment.

Research is being conducted to investigate the reason for the development of the plaques and tangles in the brain. Currently, researchers are looking at why and how these structures develop in the brain, and why certain people develop the disease and others do not.

Since the average life expectancy has increased over the past century, people are living longer with chronic illnesses and illnesses that would have killed them a century ago. It is theorized that these may be some factors that have increased the occurrence of Alzheimer's disease. It is hoped that as more research is done, more information will be uncovered to help explain and ultimately cure this devastating disease. For now, caregivers play the most important role in helping to manage the disease, whether it be by discussing changes and pursuing options with medical personnel, or by helping their loved ones maintain lifestyles that are as full and active as possible.

What we do know is that the rate of the progression for Alzheimer's disease is different for every person, and each person experiences the disease somewhat differently. Currently, when a person is diagnosed with Alzheimer's disease, their life expectancy ranges from an average of 8 to 12 years but could extend up to 20 years; however, it's quite common for people to experience the early stages of Alzheimer's disease without knowing their diagnoses.

Many caregivers say that, in retrospect, they noticed changes occurring in their loved ones for several months or even years before their diagnoses. Upon further reflection, caregivers may think that perhaps they should have said something or intervened earlier. Looking back at past events can be helpful in thinking about a timeline—for example, when did you begin noticing that changes were taking place? However, beating yourself up about what you should or could have done is not helpful. The fact that you picked up this book indicates that you are seeking guidance and that you have your loved one's best interests at heart.

Keep in mind, most people in the early or mild stages of Alzheimer's are generally able to continue living their normal lifestyle, and when trouble starts, they may initially have the ability to cover up their issues.

Of course, people have rights; these are adults who have the right to live as they wish, so as the disease progresses, if they are resistant to intervention, this aspect can become complicated for caregivers to navigate.

## EARLY MAJOR SYMPTOMS

Alzheimer's disease presents several major symptoms that most people experience. The symptoms listed here are not a comprehensive list, but are generally the most commonly reported:

- Difficulty remembering newly learned information. This is the most common early symptom, but in fact, at each stage of the disease, a variety of symptoms indicate a new problem with memory and thinking.
- Trouble remembering events.
- Confusion with relation to the passage of time.
- Difficulty finishing daily tasks at work or at home, and difficulty with focus and concentration in general.
- Difficulty with planning and problem solving. For example, a person may have difficulty with distance and spatial relationships of objects—caregivers may see their loved one having difficulty with driving. There may be reoccurring fender benders, or you may notice the corners of their bumpers are scratched and banged up. Perhaps they have gotten lost.
- An increase in poor judgment and bad decisions.

These new or recently developed behaviors, questionable decisions, and memory difficulties may have led you to suspect it's Alzheimer's disease. Perhaps a diagnosis has already been given to your loved one. Either way, many of these major symptoms indicate that a change is taking place.

## THE 7 STAGES OF COGNITIVE DECLINE

Everyone moves through the stages of Alzheimer's at a different rate over time. The progression of the disease can vary greatly, depending on factors such as the cognitive reserve and lifestyle habits of the older adult. Cognitive reserve is the older adult's ability to adapt by finding alternate ways of getting something done. This enables the person to cope with challenges and be resilient when faced with different situations, using their ability to problem-solve. This might involve things like being able to adjust plans, such as driving a different way home due to a detour, or having the capability to manage a newly prescribed medication. Cognitive reserve is an important factor that contributes to essentially protecting the brain in the early stages of Alzheimer's disease.

To briefly address lifestyle habits, the choices that people make can also impact the progression of the disease. For example, if the older adult is drinking an excessive amount of alcohol, mismanaging medications, or living an isolated, sedentary life, the brain may not have as much cognitive reserve. What's good for the heart is good for the body and the brain. Eating a diet rich in nutritionally dense foods such as leafy green vegetables and fresh fruit helps keep the body and brain healthy. Conversely, eating highly processed foods that do not have enough nutrients can contribute to poorer health. Those who live a sedentary, isolated life without exercise, purpose, or hope are prone to having less cognitive reserve than those who enjoy active lifestyles. It bears repeating that the progression of the disease looks different for each person. Generally, however, these are the stages:

### STAGE 1 – *No cognitive decline*

At this point, there is no evidence of cognitive impairment and no changes in memory, thinking, or reasoning abilities. In fact, it has been found that Alzheimer's disease begins to form in the brain approximately 20 years before any symptoms emerge or a diagnosis is given.

### STAGE 2 – *Very mild cognitive decline*

In this stage, the older adult may notice some minor problems with memory loss, and they may begin to lose or misplace items. At this stage, the person with the disease may be quite capable of explaining away these occurrences. The older adult is still doing quite well and living as they choose. Very mild cognitive decline is the beginning of the outward expression and appearance of Alzheimer's disease. Most people attribute this stage to normal age-related memory loss (see Is It Normal Aging or Alzheimer's? on page 19). The level of cognitive decline at this stage is minor.

## STAGE 3 – *Mild cognitive decline*

In this stage, the older adult may begin to have trouble explaining away their problems with memory and thinking. Family members and the soon-to-be-identified caregiver, as well as those close to the person, have started to recognize that a problem is emerging and something is just not right. The older adult may start to have increased difficulty finding the right words during conversations, organizing and planning, and remembering newly learned information. They may start to lose personal items. The cognitive decline at this stage is becoming much more evident, and the older adult is very vulnerable at this stage of the disease and from this point forward.

## STAGE 4 – *Moderate cognitive decline*

In this stage, it becomes very clear that the older adult has cognitive impairment. Problems with thinking and memory are more obvious by this stage, and the family or others close to the person are generally getting more involved. The primary caregiver starts to become a vital part of the decision-making and care coordination processes. The older adult may now have difficulty with daily tasks that they were once able to complete, such as using simple math skills, following a recipe, or writing a check. Problems with cooking may become more apparent when the older adult can no longer remember or follow the steps when trying to prepare a familiar recipe. Perhaps they are leaving the stove on, or cooking all of the liquid out of the recipe and burning the pan. At this point, safety can become a serious concern. Medication management can also become an issue, so monitoring or oversight may be needed moving forward. The level of cognitive decline is becoming a serious concern at this stage.

## STAGE 5 – *Moderate-to-severe cognitive decline*

In this stage, the older adult may need more help with many activities of daily living (ADLs). Activities of daily living include dressing, bathing, walking and moving, taking care of personal hygiene, using the bathroom, and eating. There are also instrumental activities of daily living (IADLs), which include everyday tasks such as picking out clothes that are appropriate for the season, using a telephone, managing finances, shopping for groceries, managing medications, and communicating with people. These tasks can become very challenging. There may be an increased level of confusion with severe memory loss. It's not uncommon for difficult behaviors to emerge as a result of the fear and frustration that the person may be feeling. By this stage, short-term memory is severely compromised, and a great deal of assistance may be needed to keep the loved one safe and well cared for. Interestingly, their long-term memory may still be intact at this stage. The older adult may still be able to recognize family members and reminisce about childhood and early adulthood. They may still be able to reside in their home with the assistance of support and services. By this stage of the disease, the cognitive decline creates an increased level of dependency for the older adult. The role of the caregiver becomes increasingly important in the process of coordinating the care that is needed.

## STAGE 6 – *Severe cognitive decline*

In this stage, the older adult requires constant supervision and assistance with personal care. There is an increased level of confusion and memory loss and a gap of understanding in awareness of their environment and surroundings. The older adult is unable to recall events and recognize people or places, with the exception of those who may be close by. There may be the loss of bladder and bowel control, 24/7 care is needed, and the person cannot be left alone. Assistance may be needed with feeding, and constant monitoring may be required to prevent dehydration. Personality changes, combativeness, and restlessness may accompany behavior due to the decline in cognitive functioning. For the caregiver and family, watching the deterioration of their loved one's memory and thinking abilities can be a long, devasting process to endure.

This is the final stage of this terminal disease. At this stage, people lose the ability to communicate or respond to their environment, and swallowing may become difficult. Full care is required. Ideally, by now, the caregiver and family have had time to put advanced directives in place to honor their loved one's wishes for end-of-life care.

## WHERE YOU COME IN

Alzheimer's disease is a condition that affects the entire family over time. The definition of family is fluid here, as very often, people close to an older adult may have a family of choice, such as friends, as opposed to the biological definition. Regardless of who is close by, the primary caregiver will become more active in the life of the older adult with Alzheimer's. Most often, the caregiver steps up because this older adult is very important and special to them. For other people, caregiving is thrust upon them—perhaps even by surprise and without warning.

Jane was a widow who lived alone in an apartment near friends and family in a small city. Her daughter, Terri, decided to visit for the holidays. Usually, Jane travels to her daughter's home, but this year she decided to stay home because she wasn't feeling well. Terri's brother, Billy, lived about 35 minutes away from their mom, called her twice a week, and told Terri, "Mom's fine, I talk to her all the time." Billy worked long hours and saw his mom about once a month. Terri called her mom every week and thought it was unusual that her mom didn't want to travel.

When Terri arrived at her mom's apartment, she was surprised by the condition of the apartment and her mother. Jane had always been neat and tidy—now, the garbage can was overflowing and dirty dishes were piled in the sink. In fact, the apartment smelled a little sour, and Jane needed a shower and a haircut. Terri asker her mom about the mess and why it looked like she hadn't left the apartment in many days, perhaps weeks. Jane said that she wasn't feeling well and would clean up tomorrow.

The next morning, Terri cleaned up the apartment. She was making coffee when her mother came into the kitchen and exclaimed,

"Terri, when did you get here?!" Terri said, "Ma, last night. Don't you remember?" Jane said, "Oh, that's right." They had breakfast together, and Terri suggested that her mom get cleaned up and take a shower. Jane did take a shower; however, she wanted to put the same clothes back on. Terri had her mom change into clean clothes, and they left to get a haircut. On the way to the mall, Jane asked Terri, "Where are we going?" "Ma, to the mall for your haircut," Terri reminded her. "Oh, that's right," her mom replied. Ten minutes later, she repeated, "Where are we going?" And then she asked again a few minutes later. Terri realized that something was definitely not right. Seeing her mom in the daylight, Terri realized that she looked pale and had lost weight.

It's common for adult children, friends, or relatives who haven't seen their loved one in a while to notice that changes have taken place since their previous visit. Sometimes the changes are drastic; for example, there's virtually no food in the house, they need a shower or are unkempt, the mail is stacked up, bills are unpaid. Other times, the changes can be subtle, such as bills being paid twice, medications getting mixed up, or an acute illness developing due to a fall or dehydration. Maybe you notice that your loved one has missed several appointments or that they have stopped participating in their favorite group activities.

These changes may feel like pieces of a mismatched puzzle, and you're trying to piece them together to figure out what's going on. Just as everyone experiences the progression of the disease differently, every caregiving relationship looks different as well.

## CARING FOR YOURSELF

Your personal reality of caregiving will emerge and evolve based on the needs of your loved one, so at this point it's important to be open and flexible. As a caregiver, maintaining your health and wellness is one of the most important parts of this journey. Of course, this is not to minimize your loved one, but you are the one who will play a vital part in maintaining the dignity and quality of life for your special loved one. They will need your love, patience, understanding, nonjudgmental care, and protection. And it takes energy to give all these things!

Caregiving can be rewarding, challenging, emotionally draining, and stressful. You'll most likely become a "jack of all trades," juggling the responsibilities of care while trying to live your own life. Therefore, an essential part of being an effective caregiver is making time to take care of yourself. This will be reinforced throughout the book—it's that important! You see, if you're worn out, exhausted, and overwhelmed, everyone suffers. This is preventable and doesn't need to be part of the caregiving journey.

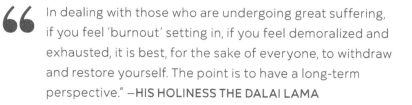 In dealing with those who are undergoing great suffering, if you feel 'burnout' setting in, if you feel demoralized and exhausted, it is best, for the sake of everyone, to withdraw and restore yourself. The point is to have a long-term perspective." —HIS HOLINESS THE DALAI LAMA

In chapter 2, we'll address next steps that begin with recognizing signs of cognitive decline in the early stages of Alzheimer's disease, learning the difference between Alzheimer's and normal aging, understanding the value of early detection, and getting to the doctor for a diagnosis.

# CHAPTER TWO

# Early Signs

### JIM'S STORY

Jim and Cathy met later in life. Cathy was 58 and Jim was 61 when they exchanged vows. After about 13 years, Cathy noticed that Jim was making mistakes in the checking account, and he had gotten lost driving on a few trips and became upset. Still, Jim had no problem driving around town, and he continued to participate in his faith community and other activities. About a year later, Cathy noticed that Jim was having difficulty speaking—first struggling to find the right words in conversations and then, later, starting to repeat himself. Then Jim lost the checkbook and couldn't find it or retrace his steps. Cathy decided to discuss her concerns with Jim's sons, Jeff and Dave. Through their discussion, Jeff shared that he, too, had become concerned about his dad recently. Dave said that when he was in town visiting, he took his dad out for lunch and he was just fine. Soon after that meeting, Cathy learned that Jim had been giving Dave money for over a year without telling her. Cathy knew it was time for Jim to see a doctor, and, in retrospect, she thought that maybe she should've had Jim checked out a few years ago.

## What to Expect

In the early stages of Alzheimer's disease—generally stages 2 and 3, also called the mild stages—most family members and caregivers won't recognize the signs of cognitive decline. For most people in the mild stages, they can manage their basic activities of daily living (ADLs), as well as most of the IADLs that are required for independent living (see page 9). We'll discuss how to recognize common signs that may occur during these early stages. Of equal importance, we'll discuss what normal aging and memory functioning may look like, as opposed to some common behaviors and symptoms that are not a normal part of the aging process. Sometimes, changes in functioning can be dismissed as "normal aging" and "just getting old." We'll challenge the belief that memory loss is a natural and normal part of the aging process. There are also some factors that can have a profound and positive impact on older adults as they age, whether or not they are experiencing memory loss, and we'll explore some ways caregivers can help.

## EARLY DETECTION

While it's important for loved ones to not beat themselves up for "not noticing sooner," the importance of early detection is worth discussing. Early detection is beneficial to the older adult with cognitive impairment, as well as to family members and caregivers. When a person experiences memory problems or increased confusion, there may be a variety of issues that could be causing this. Although there is currently no medication that can stop the progression of the disease, early detection can have a positive impact on its trajectory. Consider the following:

- There are studies that show that exercise can potentially slow the progression of the disease. Research is showing that exercise helps protect cognitive function by promoting blood flow to the brain, which nourishes the cells and neurons.
- Early detection provides the opportunity to improve one's eating habits. This will help boost overall health and wellness.
- You'll get important information sooner rather than later. The trajectory of the disease is positively impacted by the avoidance of stressful situations that can occur when you try to solve problems and make decisions without the benefit of having accurate information.
- Getting an early diagnosis can generate conversations that will help your loved one feel respected, supported, and safe.

Keeping your loved one active and engaged may help them face this frightening diagnosis with a sense of hope and purpose. When your loved one receives a diagnosis, this can actually help them address their fears and concerns, as they may have known that something was not right for a while. An interesting component to early detection is that Alzheimer's can be difficult for medical professionals to identify, because the older adult may still be able to function reasonably well for short periods of time.

## HOW THE CAREGIVER CAN HELP

A caregiver may step up and make an appointment with a doctor because they realize something is not quite right with their loved one. In this case, a common caregiver challenge can occur when they do get their loved one to the primary care office for an evaluation, and the older adult is able to talk with the doctor and answer basic questions. They are able to hold it together for a 10- or 15-minute visit. They may complete basic assessments or perform well on a short memory test. It can be tricky to detect early evidence of memory loss during these short interactions that only capture surface information. Testing in the primary care office setting is very brief and generally does not dig deeper into questioning for memory loss. This is not finding fault with the doctor or medical community. This is simply where the caregiver comes in, and it is another reason why you are so important. You can offer valuable insight and reliable information to help inform the medical provider about what you've seen, so they can put together the pieces of the puzzle to determine what may be causing the changes. Your loved one will most likely not want to admit that something is wrong with their memory and thinking. When they "perform" well for the doctor, your supplementary information and examples are critical to helping get an accurate early diagnosis.

If you can relate to this situation, this is the time to get a notebook and start taking notes about changes that you see and have seen in your loved one over time. Your real examples and documentation will help the doctor come to an accurate diagnosis, which will help your loved one receive early interventions that will benefit them in the long run.

## MILD COGNITIVE IMPAIRMENT (MCI) VS. NORMAL AGING

It's true that, as people age, more time may be needed to process complex thoughts, problem solve, or learn new things. Occasionally misplacing an item or forgetting someone's name may be quite normal and does not imply that someone has Alzheimer's disease. According to the National Institutes of Health, issues like slight forgetfulness or misplacing something from time to time can be part of the normal aging process, due to changes in the brain and body.

Normally, however, if you misplace your keys, you can retrace your steps. You know that you unlocked the door to your home with the keys and your car is parked in the driveway, so you look around the house and in your coat pockets, and eventually you find the keys. Having the ability to problem solve and retrace your steps indicates that this is not Alzheimer's disease. If you make a bad decision once in a while, that is normal; if you repeatedly make bad decisions due to poor judgment, and if you lack the insight to recognize that you've been making many poor decisions, then something else is going on.

The point of these examples is to illustrate that memory loss is not a normal part of the aging process. Cognitive decline that develops over time is not a symptom of typical aging. A normal, healthy brain is able to restore and repair the neurons that become damaged due to normal aging, illness, and everyday functioning. However, as you learned in chapter 1, in the early stages of Alzheimer's disease, the brain begins to experience irreparable interruptions in the communication among neurons.

As a caregiver, it may be helpful to get a glimpse into your loved one's changing reality. The following list of symptoms, adapted from the Alzheimer's Association's "10 Early Signs and Symptoms of Alzheimer's Disease," will help you understand some of what they might be experiencing in the early stages and decipher whether it's normal aging or something more serious:

1. **Memory loss that disrupts daily life** is one of the most common signs in the early stages. This is when the older adult may have difficulty remembering newly learned information. They may forget important dates or events, or the details associated with those events. The older adult may start asking the same question over and over or repeating themselves. There may be an increased reliance on sticky notes, alarms, calendars, or other reminders, in an effort to help remind the older adult of scheduled events, appointments, or commitments. **Examples of normal age-related changes that may not indicate Alzheimer's** include occasionally forgetting an appointment but remembering it later and mixing up two different appointments when there are many of them in the calendar.

2. **Challenges in planning or solving problems** may develop in the early stages. Some people may have trouble working with numbers or keeping track of monthly bills. They may have difficulty following a plan or even a familiar recipe. If you are a loved one, you've watched this person plan and cook the holiday family dinner your entire life. You realize that, recently, this has become a daunting process for them. They get flustered and irritable in the days leading up to the event. Important dishes are omitted and others may not be cooked properly. **An example of a normal age-related change that may not indicate Alzheimer's** is when an older adult forgets to heat up a dish in the oven, but remembers it when they see it in the refrigerator.

3. **Difficulty completing familiar tasks** can be another early sign of Alzheimer's disease. Just as your loved one is having difficulty planning a family meal, on a more detailed level, you realize that although your loved one has made a familiar recipe for 40 or 50 years, this has become a challenging process. If it's marinara

sauce, maybe the olive oil, spices, and garlic are left out. If it's their awesome mac and cheese, perhaps the macaroni is added uncooked or, instead of cheese, a block of butter is added. Perhaps there's no water in the coffee maker or no recollection of having turned the coffee maker on. Or maybe your loved one is getting frustrated trying to start the lawn mower or tractor, and you notice that the fuel tank is completely empty. **An example of a normal age-related change that may not indicate Alzheimer's** is when your loved one is super busy, distracted, or generally worn out, and just forgets to add water or an ingredient to a recipe.

4.  **Confusion with time or place** can be another early symptom of Alzheimer's disease. The Alzheimer's Association states that people with the disease can lose track of the passage of time, dates, and even seasons. The older adult may have difficulty understanding that an event is not happening immediately. Your loved one may forget where they are or how they got there. They may not understand that an appointment is planned several weeks or months ahead and that missing an appointment can waste valuable time, as they'll now have to wait to be seen again. Confusion with time and place can be tricky for the caregiver to identify in the early stages; the older adult may still be able to somewhat cover up this emerging problem. **An example of a normal age-related change that may not indicate Alzheimer's** is when an older adult encounters a detour and gets lost, but is still able to find their way home.

5.  **Trouble understanding visual images and spatial relationships** is a lesser-known sign of Alzheimer's disease. This can interfere with your loved one's ability to read and understand words and text. The caregiver may see that their loved one is reading the newspaper, but they might not realize that their loved one is unable to comprehend what they are seeing. Very often, difficulty driving emerges with the progression of the disease. The caregiver may notice that the older adult is having fender benders and bumping into curbs or light posts. The outer corners of the older adult's bumpers may be scratched, dented, or banged up. The older adult may have developed trouble with their depth percep-

tion. **An example of a normal age-related change that does not indicate Alzheimer's** is experiencing vision changes due to a medical condition such as cataracts.

6.  **New problems with words in speaking or writing** can develop as a sign and symptom of Alzheimer's disease. The older adult may stop in the middle of a conversation and be at a loss for words or start to repeat themselves. They may also struggle to find the correct word for an item, such as calling a bird "a flying thing" or calling spaghetti "that long, stringy stuff you eat." For the caregiver, this can be an outward sign that something may be wrong with their loved one. **An example of a normal age-related change that may not indicate Alzheimer's** is forgetting the name of a bird, but calling it a bird and then recalling or looking up the name later on.

7.  **Misplacing things and losing the ability to retrace steps** is a very common sign of Alzheimer's disease. Your loved one may put an item in an unusual place and then be unable to retrace their steps to find it. They may put a credit card in the freezer under the ice cube tray or put their purse in the oven for safekeeping. Caregivers or others may be wrongfully accused of stealing things or hiding their loved one's items. This may occur more frequently over time. **An example of a normal age-related change that may not indicate Alzheimer's** is when an older adult misplaces their keys or glasses, but is then able to retrace their steps to find them.

8.  **Decreased or poor judgment** may emerge as a result of Alzheimer's disease. The older adult may start to make some bad decisions. This can include giving away money to family members, strangers, or telemarketers. Or, perhaps they allow someone into their home who doesn't belong there or pay in advance for a home improvement project that never gets started or that they really don't need or can't afford. Another outward sign that changes may be occurring is that your loved one loses interest in self-care. Their personal appearance may start to change; perhaps you've noticed that they aren't showering as often or that they are wearing the same clothes all of the time.

They may have always been well groomed, but now you notice that they are looking unkempt. **An example of a normal age-related change that may not indicate Alzheimer's** is when an older adult decides to skip an occasional shower, but still puts on fresh clothes and brushes their teeth.

9. **Withdrawal from work or social activities** may occur, as the older adult may become hesitant to participate in familiar activities or groups. They may have difficulty watching or following their favorite sports team, or perhaps they lose interest in hobbies that they once enjoyed. The caregiver may notice that their loved one has begun to isolate themselves and avoid familiar situations. **An example of a normal age-related change that may not indicate Alzheimer's** is when an older adult feels worn out from family or work obligations, so they decide to skip an occasional event.

10. **Changes in mood or personality** can also be early signs of Alzheimer's disease. Personality changes can be caused by feelings of confusion, fear, anxiety, suspicion, or depression and can cause your loved one to communicate and act very differently. They may become easily upset or anxious in places and situations that are not in their comfort zone, and this could be very much out of character for them. For a caregiver, this can be distressing to watch, because you may not yet have put all of the pieces of the puzzle together as your loved one changes. **An example of a normal age-related change that may not indicate Alzheimer's** is when an older adult seems mildly uncomfortable in a new environment or when a routine is interrupted.

It's important to remember that every person experiences the progression of Alzheimer's disease differently. Older adults may display one or more of these early signs, but they can differ based upon your loved one's personality, medical history, and many other factors.

Imagine that your daughter is telling you about a birthday party that you both attended yesterday. She's talking about the people and the gifts and the cake, and yet, in your head, you're not quite sure whose birthday it was, having no recollection of the party. In fact, you're pretty sure it never happened. You know that your daughter wouldn't lie, but she's wrong.

Likewise, do you know how it feels to wake up groggy and disoriented from a minor surgical procedure for which you're given a sedative? Picture yourself at the exact moment you wake up—now, you are immediately expected to get up, find your clothes that you left in the pre-op room, get dressed, identify and thank the lead nurse in the recovery room, and then drive home. You may still feel unclear, your judgment is off, and you may not even remember why you were there. For a moment, think about how you would feel trying to manage all of that on your own when you weren't thinking clearly. Your loved one may feel like that when they go to the grocery store, make dinner, or balance their checkbook after paying the bills. It can be scary, frustrating, and embarrassing.

## What to Say

1. **Be inclusive.** In the early stages of the disease, communication will vary based on the needs of the older adult. Your loved one will most likely be quite able to participate in meaningful conversations, but they may have difficulty comprehending new information or understanding complex situations or explanations. **Try not to make assumptions or exclude your loved one from conversations.** If problems emerge with communication, work together to find a solution to help ease their discomfort and embarrassment. If you're at the doctor's office and you start speaking to the nurse about your loved one while they are present, be sure to include them in the conversation.

2. **Listen to your loved one.** Give them time to share their thoughts, feelings, and needs. Try to be patient and allow them the chance to communicate with you.

3. **Take your time.** When caregivers are busy, it can be a challenge to slow down and listen, but a patient caregiver can really help put their loved one at ease.

4. **Ask questions.** Try to determine what your loved one is comfortable doing and what they might need help with. This can be awkward at first, and you may not get an honest answer. Most people don't want to admit that they need help. You can always just say that you're available to help as needed.

5. **Give your loved one time to respond.** More time may be needed to process a conversation and respond. Although it can be tempting to interrupt them, try to be patient and offer support that's not judgmental or condescending.

6. **Admit when you're not sure what to say.** Treat your loved one with dignity and respect. When they say something unusual or out of character, instead of reacting in a negative or judgmental way, tell them, "I'm not really sure what to say right now."

7. **Laugh.** Benjamin Franklin is quoted as saying, "Trouble knocked at the door, but, hearing laughter, hurried away." Sometimes laughter really is the best medicine, and it can help bring people together and lift their spirits when it's most needed.

8. **Keep your cool.** When your loved one is repeating themselves, it may be best to just listen, rather than insist on correcting them. If the older adult is getting agitated, upset, or overwhelmed, the repetition may increase. This situation can be made even worse if you, as the caregiver, constantly correct them. If you're tempted to say, "Mom I told you five times already—you're driving me crazy," try to catch yourself and realize that this will not help the situation. However, you're only human, and sometimes you just need to step away when you're out of patience—that's okay, too!

# What to Do

The early stages of Alzheimer's disease can be confusing for everyone involved. One day, the older adult appears to be fine; the next day, they're not. On a Monday in June they may think it's September 30th, and the very next day, they may know the date and season without a problem. You may realize that unpredictable occurrences like these have been going on for a few years, and they are now happening more frequently. It's time to take action and get your loved one to a doctor, preferably a neurologist. If you feel comfortable doing so, talk with your loved one about what they're feeling. They may open up to you and provide valuable insight that you can present to the doctor. Or, enlist the help of another trusted relative or friend with whom your loved one may be willing to share some of what they've been feeling and experiencing.

## SEEKING A DIAGNOSIS

A caregiver may be eager to get a diagnosis so they can start doing what they can to help with this situation. However, the older adult may not be quite as ready to face the situation or even believe that anything is wrong with them. Facing the reality of memory loss can be terrifying and overwhelming for everyone involved. It's important not to underestimate the impact of making such a life-changing decision. When and if your loved one does decide to see a doctor, this means they are acknowledging the fact that something is wrong with them.

Unlike most cancers, diabetes, and other illnesses, a diagnosis of Alzheimer's disease indicates that something is wrong with your loved one's brain and that, ultimately, they will lose their ability to make decisions for themselves. However, with an early diagnosis, your loved one will still be able to plan in order to have their decisions honored and their wishes respected. If your loved one refuses to see their doctor or a neurologist, here are some talking points you can use to start the discussion:

* Early detection gives us time to learn about the diagnosis and what to expect.

- Early diagnosis allows you the opportunity to make choices about treatment options, including potential access to clinical trials and research studies.
- Diagnosis gives us the opportunity to build a care team and learn about support services.

## WHAT TO ASK THE DOCTOR

First thing: Get a notebook! Track your loved one's changes in this notebook, and write down your questions in advance to prepare for the appointment. Most importantly, plan to bring this notebook to every doctor's visit.

Start by making an appointment for your loved one to be seen by a primary care physician (PCP). This may be a doctor with whom they have a long-standing relationship, or perhaps it's a new doctor. They may see another healthcare professional, such as a physician's assistant or nurse practitioner. Some primary care doctors and staff are comfortable treating patients who have memory loss, while others prefer to make a referral to a neurologist to make the specialized diagnosis.

Once you are at the doctor's office, it's important to be both honest and thorough about what's going on. Decide ahead of time if you have the ability and courage to speak in front of your loved one. Some caregivers request to speak privately to the medical professional during the office visit. This can be a tough decision to make, because it may feel disrespectful telling the doctor about all of the troubles your loved one is having. Whether you decide to speak privately or in front of your loved one, it's important to be candid. You may want to tell your loved one that you're being honest, and that, although this is very upsetting, their health, safety, and wellness is the most important priority right now. Show kindness, love, and patience to your loved one and yourself; this is a tough visit for both of you.

- Acknowledgment of the situation means that we have more time to make future plans regarding financial and legal matters, as well as decisions about healthcare and long-term planning.

For the caregiver, care partner, spouse, and family members, the benefits of an early diagnosis include the following:

Go in with a list of examples of your concerns. *For example: When Mom is cooking, she forgets ingredients, and we just found out that she has left the stove on several times.* Or: *My husband has misplaced the credit card four times. We've replaced it, but he keeps losing things and can't find them.* List specific changes in behaviors, when they occur, how long they last, and what seems to trigger them. Take note if they're anxious, moody, crying, depressed, or angry. You can give this list to the nurse upon arrival.

Be brave and inquisitive. Ask the doctor why there may be difficulty with memory and thinking that has developed over time. You can ask if it could be Alzheimer's disease, or if there is something else that could be causing these changes. Did your loved one develop these changes suddenly or overnight? When talking to the doctor, ask direct questions (or bring someone with you who will) to ensure that you get your answers and that the doctor has all of the information needed to make a well-informed diagnosis.

It's important to tell the doctor about changes in mood, behaviors, or situations that help tell your loved one's story and explain that these are significant changes—real reasons for concern. If you're told that this is a normal part of aging, perhaps you need a second opinion, preferably from a neurologist. Don't accept an opinion that these changes are unimportant, and don't allow your concerns to be dismissed or brushed off. Clearly, these changes in your loved one have brought you to the doctor's office for help. Be persistent in getting a diagnosis, because having an accurate diagnosis will best serve this special person and all those involved. Visit chapter 4 (page 53) for more information on getting an Alzheimer's diagnosis.

- The opportunity to learn what to expect and what to address, such as current symptoms, challenges, behavioral changes, and safety issues associated with the disease's progression
- Time for those involved in the care plan to develop their own support system to help them throughout this difficult disease
- The ability to make more informed decisions regarding levels or types of care that may be needed as the disease progresses
- An opened door to discussions about advanced directives and end-of-life wishes, which will ensure that the older adult is provided with the best and most personalized care possible

When denial is firmly set in and your loved one refuses to see a doctor, they do have the right to refuse. This is an adult with rights, and you cannot force them to get a diagnosis. If this does happen, you can call your loved one's doctor and leave a message indicating that you're concerned about your loved one. By law, the doctor cannot even acknowledge that your loved one is a patient in that practice. However, you can inform the doctor of your concerns, then immediately follow up with a letter giving concrete examples of why you're concerned about your loved one. For example: *Dad keeps getting lost while driving, and he keeps forgetting to take his medication.* Or, *Dad is having trouble finding the right words for things, and he's anxious and upset lately. We've noticed the changes in our dad for about a year now. He's refusing to talk about it, and we're concerned about his safety and well-being.* Now, the condition is documented with the physician. You may have to wait for an answer, but hopefully not. If you don't get a response or some indication that this is being addressed, write another letter—be courteous but persistent.

Your advocacy, persistence, and concern will positively impact your loved one's life and well-being. They will need protection when their reasoning and judgment become impaired, as they'll be highly vulnerable to scams, getting lost, and other harmful situations.

Do not give up—even if your loved one won't budge, you can still be of tremendous help and influence. If you can't get them to the doctor's office, think about a person whom your loved one will listen to. Enlist the help of that person, whether it's a trusted friend of the family or an authoritative figure they respect, such as a leader of their faith community, to help encourage them to get to a doctor's office. If they are a retired firefighter, for example, enlist the help of a fellow firefighter.

Some families use a "good cop/bad cop" approach. This is not stated with disrespect for police officers; rather, it's a creative method that involves two people who work together to effect a change—one with a gentle, supportive approach, and one with a "You've gotta toughen up and do this" approach—with both approaches seeking the same outcome. This isn't about coercion or use of force. It's about persistence and a willingness to try multiple strategies to get your loved one to a doctor's office.

Despite any apprehensions one may have about facing this reality, getting an accurate diagnosis for your loved one can be one of the best steps you can take to improve the quality of life for your loved one and yourself as the caregiver.

## SELF-CARE

As a caregiver, this may all be new to you. Be gentle with yourself—this journey can be scary and overwhelming. On some levels, it can also be a rewarding experience that draws you closer to your loved one. You are making difficult decisions, though, and this can be very stressful. Just as it's important to get an early diagnosis, it's equally important to remember, from the beginning, if possible, to take care of yourself. Keeping yourself physically and emotionally healthy and well will help you better manage this unpredictable chapter in your life. And, of course, your loved one needs you to be healthy and present! If you're worn out, exhausted, and totally stressed, it can make a challenging situation worse than it needs to be. You are very special and deserve to be healthy and well.

 Compassion and tolerance are not a sign of weakness, but a sign of strength." –HIS HOLINESS THE DALAI LAMA

## JUST ONE THING

If there's just one message that you take from this book as your concern grows for that special loved one, let it be this: Be gentle with yourself; be kind to yourself. Life may have thrown you a curveball, taking you down a path that you had never anticipated. In it all, celebrate the small victories, find a reason to laugh every day, and do one small act of kindness **just for you** every day. If you had 5 or 10 minutes all to yourself, what would you do? Listen to music, read something inspirational, plan some quiet time with your partner? Text funny emojis to your best friend? Maybe you just want to watch a few lighthearted videos on the Internet, or grab the latest fashion magazine and a cup of coffee or tea and get lost in the beautiful styles. Shoot some hoops, take a quick walk around the block, breathe in the fresh air, practice gratitude ... the list is endless. Whatever speaks to your heart, do it as often as you can.

 If your compassion does not include yourself, it is incomplete." —JACK KORNFIELD

PART TWO

# EARLY AND MIDDLE STAGES

The early and middle stages of Alzheimer's constitute the longest part of the disease. For most people, this is when stage 3 (mild cognitive decline), stage 4 (moderate cognitive decline), and stage 5 (moderate to severe cognitive decline) develop. For you, it probably means that your life has changed drastically, you've become more involved as a caregiver, and the future feels somewhat uncertain. This part of the book will cover in detail what you can expect during this time of transition. I'll also offer some practical tips to address the most common situations that can occur during this part of the journey, as you become more involved in planning and caring for your loved one.

# CHAPTER THREE

# Early Memory Loss

## SAMUEL'S STORY

Selma and Samuel have been married for 40 years. Samuel is retired, but Selma still works part-time as a clerk, with plans to retire in three years. She had to shift her employment status from full-time to part-time when Samuel was diagnosed with Alzheimer's disease. Selma realized that Samuel could no longer stay home alone all day without anyone checking on him. He had gotten lost driving, and his license had been taken away. More recently, he went for a walk and was gone for about five hours when a former coworker, Gerry, finally found Samuel sitting on a park bench near his old office. He had walked four miles "to work" in the rain without his coat, hat, or glasses. Gerry tracked down Selma at work, and she rushed over to pick up Samuel, frantic and worried sick. Gerry explained that this was the second time he had run into Samuel near the office—the first time they briefly talked, and Samuel found his way home. Gerry initially didn't know that Samuel was no longer driving, and he now understood that there was a problem with his friend's memory. Selma also discovered that Samuel wasn't taking his medications properly, nor eating lunch.

Now that Selma has changed from full-time to part-time, Samuel stays home alone for just a few hours each morning. Selma makes breakfast, gives Samuel his medication, and then works from 9 a.m. to 1 p.m. This plan has worked quite well for almost two years, but as the disease has progressed further into the moderate-to-severe stage, Selma's discovering that it's no longer safe for Samuel to be alone. However, she can't retire for another year, or her benefits will be substantially reduced. Her retirement income was already reduced by 14 percent when she cut her hours back, and she can't afford to lose any more benefits. She needs to develop a new plan of care for Samuel to help her get through the next year, until she can retire.

## What to Expect

As the cognitive decline progresses and your loved one has more difficulty with memory loss and confusion, you may find your life filled with unexpected situations. There may be a new sense of shame and perhaps denial, in that your loved one may not want to disclose their diagnosis or let others know that there is a very serious problem going on. A new, higher level of caregiving is unfolding, and in this chapter, we'll walk through some of the most common challenges and difficult situations that you'll likely encounter. I'd say this is about what to expect moving forward, but to sum it up, it may be more fitting to say, *expect the unexpected*. As Alzheimer's disease progresses, this experience can look different for every person. You'll benefit from surrounding yourself with supportive people and getting the most up-to-date and accurate information to help guide you. Be open to learning all you can about the disease. Expect that you may feel off balance or overwhelmed at times. During these times, it's important to continue being as patient and nonjudgmental as you can with your loved one, and of course, to be kind to yourself as well.

### MEMORY LOSS AND CONFUSION

In the early and middle or moderate stages of Alzheimer's disease, more obvious changes will emerge in your loved one's personality and functioning. You'll begin to witness greater difficulty in their ability to perform routine tasks, such as calling the pharmacy for medication refills or keeping track of appointments. They will probably experience increased difficulty in following a set of instructions, such as: *Get a turkey sandwich out of the refrigerator, pour a glass of milk, and be sure to take the correct medication with lunch.* A seemingly simple process may become too complicated for your loved one to complete. This is typically when driving becomes dangerous for the older adult. Tasks and habits that your loved one has done "on autopilot" for many years will become more challenging as the disease progresses. Just as Samuel, from the previous story, could no longer manage his medications and make himself lunch, your loved one may suddenly not be able to manage certain tasks that they had no problems doing for quite a while. If your loved one has always done the grocery shopping, this process may become positively overwhelming for them, due to the complexity of thoughts and problem-solving involved.

As forgetfulness increases, your loved one may lose the ability to recall important information such as their address or phone number, and this can put them at risk if they get lost. Becoming lost and disoriented is very common for people with Alzheimer's disease, so your loved one may need more supervision to prevent them from wandering or getting lost. They may lose the ability to recall personal and family history, and forgetting the names of family members is also very common. They may have problems recalling words or details about special events, such as weddings, births, or funerals—things you know they would be able to remember if they didn't have Alzheimer's disease. There may be increased confusion about time and place—not knowing where they are and having difficulty with the times and sequences of when events took place.

## EMOTIONS

During this part of the disease progression, your loved one is experiencing many losses, with the main focus generally being on the loss of independence. Encourage your loved one to be as independent as possible, while remaining safe. It is devastating to face the losses of freedom and the ability to make decisions. Your loved one might be overwhelmed and frightened, and they may not have the ability to articulate how this makes them feel. This can cause feelings of frustration and impatience. They may feel the need to exert their authority by digging in their heels and refusing any help or suggestions.

As the disease progresses, your loved one will have trouble managing their emotions when they surface, due to the changes in their brain. Alzheimer's disease can cause strong emotional reactions to minor problems, such as crying, shouting, or refusing to participate in an activity. Emotional responses can be confusing to the people who witness them. You may wonder how to recognize or understand the meanings behind the triggers of these emotional episodes, as your loved one tries to make sense of the world around them. You can offer reassurance by staying calm and not being judgmental or critical in your response to their actions. Your gentle support and love can greatly ease these stressful situations.

## DEPRESSION AND APATHY

As Alzheimer's disease continues to impact your loved one, they may experience a loss of interest, or apathy, when it comes to activities they once enjoyed. This is very common, as impairments in memory and thinking can make it difficult to fully participate in familiar and pleasurable activities. Apathy can also look like depression, and depression is also very common in this stage of the disease.

To distinguish, apathy is a state of withdrawal that, for people with Alzheimer's disease, can result from a lack of confidence in their abilities. To the outsider, this looks like a loss of motivation and interest in hobbies and activities, especially those that require planning and sequencing tasks. The more complicated the task, the less likely your loved one will be able to manage that hobby or activity. Even if they've done this activity their entire adult life, apathy causes the lack of interest that often looks like a loss of energy or excitement about those pleasurable hobbies or activities. If your loved one is feeling apathetic, they may react with indifference and detachment to feelings, situations, and even the people around them.

Isolation and apathy caused by Alzheimer's disease can lead to depression. In fact, about 40 percent of all people with Alzheimer's disease also develop depression. As you can well imagine, that can really negatively impact your loved one. The good news is, depression can be treated successfully with the help of your loved one's doctor. Watch out for and don't dismiss the symptoms that may emerge—depression is a common co-occurring condition that, when not treated properly, can greatly worsen your loved one's quality of life.

Some symptoms of depression mimic symptoms of apathy. These are:

- Social isolation
- Loss of interest in pleasurable activities

However, additional symptoms that may point to depression include:

- Changes in appetite
- Disruption in sleep
- Irritability
- Fatigue or loss of energy
- Feelings of hopelessness, loss, sadness, or excessive guilt
- Thoughts of suicide and death

Although this is very rare, if your loved one talks about suicide or ending it all—comments like *"Why bother to live?"* or *"Why should I care about my life?"*—treat these statements seriously, and call the doctor immediately! Ask your loved one if they have a plan for how they may take their own life, and try your best not to panic in the moment. Remember that the changes in your loved one's brain are causing disruptions in their thinking and processing of thoughts and emotions. Redirect your loved one in the moment by offering them some food or a cup of coffee, or getting them out of the house for a car ride—this may interrupt the negative thoughts. Still, do call the doctor and stay with your loved one until you're sure that they will be safe and not harm themselves.

Depression is treatable with medication management in partnership with the doctor. This, along with helping your loved one participate in pleasurable and meaningful activities that are appropriate for their abilities, will provide hope and satisfaction for your loved one and reduce feelings of depression. It's also important for your loved one to stay connected to people who are part of a trusted, loving, and nonjudgmental support system.

## SOCIALIZING

Perhaps you've noticed that your loved one has been isolating themself and not participating in activities or social situations. They may become moody or irritable when prompted to go to an event or leave their home. Social withdrawal is common for people in the early stages of Alzheimer's, as they have increased difficulties functioning outside of their homes or in unfamiliar environments. Socializing also reveals that your loved one has developed deficits due to the disease. Think about how you can help your loved one interact with friends who understand what is happening. Perhaps they can take your loved one out; understanding friends will be flexible if the plan needs to be adjusted or changed. There may be local opportunities for your loved one to attend outings specifically for people with memory loss. Local adult day programs can also engage your loved one in pleasurable, meaningful activities.

## CHANGES IN SLEEP

Almost every person with Alzheimer's disease will at some point experience changes in their sleep patterns. They may begin sleeping a lot during the day and be up most of the night. Alzheimer's disease can disrupt the sleep cycle, causing your loved one to have difficulty staying asleep at night. This can be positively exhausting for caregivers. However, by watching for and taking note of any changes in your loved one's sleep patterns, you can provide essential information to their doctor to help regulate sleep and prevent additional related issues from occurring, such as nighttime wandering.

If sleep disturbances occur, call the doctor for suggestions to help solve this problem. Medications can help, as well as strategies to keep your loved one engaged and busy during the day. Can they go to a senior center for lunch or spend part of the day in an adult day program? When your loved one has busy activities during the day, this will promote better sleep at night. Be sure to keep track in your notebook of when the sleep issues started, how often these issues occur, and what your loved one is doing at night. That way, you'll have accurate information for the doctor when you call or attend the next appointment.

## CHANGES IN PERSONALITY

As the disease progresses, you may notice profound changes in your loved one's personality and behaviors. Some of the behaviors that emerge can be very disturbing for the caregiver and the family. The older adult coping with Alzheimer's may even become suspicious of you and others around them, and they may make unfounded accusations about people stealing or hiding things from them. They may have started hoarding things such as food, napkins, tissues (clean or used), and other items that should be thrown away. The disease progression causes these changes in your loved one's personality, so try to understand that this disease is destroying their brain and your loved one is only trying to adapt. Ironically, for some people who may not have been very pleasant or nice previously in their life, the disease can cause changes in their brain that result in a more positive disposition. Others who may have been kind and pleasant throughout their life are now acting mean and nasty. Alzheimer's disease causes changes in personality—sometimes for the worse, sometimes for the better. Try to remember that this is out of their control, and continue to be supportive and nonjudgmental in your approach and interactions.

## HOARDING

According to the Alzheimer's Association, an individual's propensity to hoard, rummage, and hide items often stems from memory loss, mental confusion, disorientation, and impaired judgment.

Hoarding is more likely to occur in the early part of the middle stages of the disease, and it may be linked with the older adult's feelings that they are losing control of their life. These behaviors may be an attempt to rebalance with a sense of security. As the disease progresses, hoarding may get worse, because the individual no longer recognizes their family, caregiver, or environment, and is driven to search for items they believe were stolen or hidden from them.

If your loved one starts to exhibit bizarre behaviors such as hoarding, it's time to reach out to the doctor. Keeping your loved safe is the first priority, but helping them *feel* safe is also important.

## DRIVING

When your loved one is no longer capable of driving, taking away the keys and informing your loved one of this determination are two of the worst tasks in your caregiver journey. Actually, if you're the only person the older adult trusts, you may not want to be the one to tell them. Many physicians and health providers are willing to tell an older adult when they are no longer safe to drive, and their authority tends to be respected. Think about others who can be "the bad guy" instead of you. Perhaps a member or leader in your loved one's faith community or a friend of the family would be willing to step up. Another option is to look in your area for organizations that provide driving evaluations. These evaluations are sometimes available at hospitals that have rehabilitation services. Your county office for aging would have that information, as would your physician. Driver evaluations are often covered by insurance, but a physician referral is generally required. Putting this job in the hands of a third party is best—that way, the caregiver is not to blame for this devastating loss to the older adult.

Another strategy is to disable the vehicle by disconnecting the battery and declaring that the car broke down and needs to be repaired. Then, remove the vehicle and do not replace it. If your loved one is capable of having a car repaired or getting behind the wheel of another vehicle, reach out to the physician and ask them for help. The family can also make a report to their state's department of motor vehicles to request that their loved one's license be revoked. Generally, the process goes like this: The older adult is notified, then a driver evaluation is given, medical records are requested, and a hearing can be scheduled to address the situation.

Keeping your loved one safe is a priority, and so is keeping other people safe from a driver who should no longer be on the road. Difficult conversations and tough decisions are parts of the caregiver role that most people cannot imagine or anticipate. These can be some of the most stressful moments you will face as a caregiver. When you're carrying these burdens, take extra time to care and do kind things for yourself. It's important for you to remember that you're doing an honorable thing, even if it doesn't feel so great at the moment.

Keep in mind that having the keys taken away is a very common event for those suffering with Alzheimer's. Eventually, everyone with the disease will lose the ability to drive—this is a progressive neurological disease that interferes with all aspects of daily living.

## SAFETY

When it comes to safety, consider what is at risk, then pick your battles carefully! When your loved one insists on making the coffee in the morning but always leaves the coffee pot on, replace the coffee maker with a unit that has an automatic shut-off feature. Then, you won't have to argue or worry about it being left on. If they insist on wearing clothes that don't match, try to let that one go, as long as they are dressed appropriately for the weather. Wearing a heavy coat in the summer can be dangerous to their health. Offer a lighter coat and remove the heavy winter coat to a back closet until cooler weather returns.

The time to pick a battle is when safety is jeopardized and your loved one could be harmed. "Sorry, my dear, your safety must come first." Yes, your loved one will be very upset with you. As the caregiver, this can be difficult. Being a caregiver is hard; you're making difficult and unpopular decisions to protect your loved one, but that is always the right thing to do. The secret to surviving this part is to encourage your loved one to make decisions for themselves that will not put them at risk for harm. You can even empower them by asking their opinion or seeking their advice on things. Even if you don't follow their advice, you'll have made them feel like their thoughts are valued.

If you're a perfectionist, the balancing act of picking your battles may mean that you'll have to let some things be imperfect in order to respect the dignity of your loved one. If you can handle these sorts of compromises, you can take it one step further by following a direction with a question. If you've decisively taken your mom's coat away because it's July, ask her opinion on your outfit, or ask her if she'd like to walk down this block or that block with you. Picking your battles and including your loved one in decision-making when possible can have a positive impact on your loved one's quality of life.

For the older adult, going through the moderate stage of Alzheimer's disease can be frightening, disorienting, and embarrassing—it can feel like their world has changed forever. Sadly, it has. The brain of the older adult is actually shrinking in size. As the brain shrinks, the connections between the neurons are damaged and the brain can no longer function at a normal level. Their lifelong capacity to think, process, and remember has been interrupted, and thoughts cannot be completed. Medically, they may not even recognize the feelings of being thirsty or hungry or having a fever. Take a moment to imagine yourself in their shoes—you wouldn't know where to find a shoe, or you'd put on a shoe that doesn't fit properly. You once loved to sit on the porch and relax with a book or magazine, but now you don't want to go outside because you can't remember the pleasure of sitting on the porch. This is when you as the caregiver can offer comfort and support. Go ahead and invite your loved one to sit on the porch with you—and smile, because you know this makes your loved one happy.

# What to Say

In the middle or moderate stages of the disease, communication will most likely become more challenging for your loved one. Losing the ability to speak in complete sentences or to articulate needs can naturally cause frustration and agitation for the older adult. In this case, it can be helpful to keep conversations and communication clear, concise, and direct. At the same time, it's important not to speak to the older adult as if they are a child. Good examples of appropriate messages include:

*"Mom, how about a glass of water? I'm thirsty—let's have some together."*

*"Dad, I like your socks—they don't match. You must have another pair just like 'em in the drawer." (And smile because you just made a joke, and it's okay if the socks don't match.)*

*"Dad, Dr. Jones said that driving isn't safe anymore. It was the doctor's decision, not mine. I'm so sorry that you're upset. At the next appointment, let's ask Dr. Jones again about it." (Move the car out of the driveway or disable it.) "Dad, the car is broken again—we'll have it looked at."*

*"Mom, let's have lunch; a sandwich sounds good today. I love grilled cheese—is that okay with you?"*

*"Mom, I just made a grilled cheese; I can't finish it. Would you like half?*

Even as the disease progresses, the person with Alzheimer's will know when someone is patronizing or speaking to them like a child. Instead, try using a calm voice, and speak just a little slower than you normally would. Speaking fast and giving them too much information at one time can make your loved one feel overwhelmed and anxious, and can even trigger difficult behaviors in response to the stress of communication. Here are some suggestions for good communication:

- Talk to your loved one in a quiet environment with minimal distractions. Whenever possible, turn off the TV and turn down the radio.
- Ask yes/no questions, and use gestures and nonverbal cues to help your loved one understand what is being asked of them.
- Maintain eye contact to show that you're listening and interested in what they are saying.
- Bend down or grab a chair to sit down and communicate at eye level, rather than leaning over them or talking down at them, which can make your loved one feel like you're being overbearing or bossy.
- Give the person time to respond after you've asked them a question. Be patient and offer reassurance; try not to be too quick in finding the right word for your loved one, and give them a chance to answer your question in their words.
- Resist the urge to argue with or criticize your loved one as they struggle to communicate with you. When your patience is stretched to the limit and your loved one is being difficult

or obstinate, yelling, arguing, or trying to orient them to your reality only escalates the situation. Meet your loved one where they are, be gentle and calm, and step away for some deep breaths whenever you need to.

## What to Do

It's clear that being a caregiver is not an easy task, and you're hopefully all in on this for the duration. Give yourself a hug—you deserve it. Now, it's time to think about things you can do to make this journey a little easier on you and your loved one.

Surrounding yourselves with an environment that is safe and comfortable is key. First, you'll want to simplify your physical environment. Try not to move furniture unless it's absolutely necessary, such as for safety reasons. This will help keep your loved one oriented to the space and reduce tripping hazards.

You can also simplify your emotional environment. Try your best to have a routine or structure throughout the day. Offering some level of predictability will help make your loved one feel safe. Even though they have problems with memory and thinking, a routine is helpful for the caregiver and essential for the older adult.

If your loved one is hoarding or hiding food in their closet, you as the caregiver know that the food must be taken out to prevent mice or bugs from getting in the house or apartment. A little creativity may be needed for this one. You can clean out the mess when your loved one is out, but they may just start to collect food again. They may also start putting it somewhere else, so keep on the lookout for evidence of this habit. You could replace the food you find in areas where food should not be stored with cleaned, empty boxes of similar food—this can prevent infestation. Depending on your loved one's level of cognitive functioning, such creative thinking may be needed to protect their safety, health, and wellness. Explaining why you're removing the food may only escalate the situation; rather, it may be best to quietly keep them safe through clever problem solving.

Make lists to help keep everyone organized. You can put these lists in places where your loved one will see them. For example, put a sign on the door, above the doorknob, that reads:

- Get your keys.
- Close the door behind you.

A note by the phone might read:

- Jon's [or my] number is ***-***-****.
- I'll be home at 5:00.

A note on the refrigerator could read:

- Sandwich in fridge for lunch.
- Glass of tea is next to the sink.

You can also try to make things easy to find, such as always placing TV remotes in the basket on the coffee table. Predictability can contribute to a flow that works.

Within the daily routine, you can help your loved one feel like their opinions are valued. Some safe activities include letting them pick out their own clothes, make decisions about what to eat, and choose what activities they'll do (all with your supervision). Avoid choice overload; your loved one may become overwhelmed. Instead, set out two outfits for your loved one so they can pick which one to wear. For breakfast, let them pick the type of cereal or toast they want to eat. Encouraging them to make decisions and have some sense of control when they are slowly losing control of their world is a powerful way to make your loved one feel respected and dignified. Additionally, as a caregiver, giving them a few choices can help you minimize distractions and avoid arguments over having no choices or too many choices. A predictable and peaceful structure will help everyone involved feel safe and secure. Finally, try to be patient. It may take them longer to do things. When you have plans or an appointment with them, figure in the extra time they'll need to get ready.

## WHAT TO ASK THE DOCTOR

The doctor can prove a valuable resource as the situation is changing, whether your loved one is acting differently, having difficulty sleeping, or experiencing other problems. Preparing for the office visit is time well spent; write down questions or concerns in your notebook beforehand. Mark the dates and times of any unusual or new behaviors. List all current medications, supplements, and vitamins that your loved one is taking, including the dosages. Here are some great questions to ask:

- What can we expect about changes in behaviors?
- Can depression or anxiety be treated at this stage? Will they test for that?
- Can they participate in a clinical trial? We would be interested in participating in research if my loved one qualifies. (Many neurologists and hospitals provide research opportunities and are often recruiting for clinical trials. If your doctor does not have a connection to any research studies or similar programs, ask if there are other opportunities to participate in your region.)
- Are there any experimental medications that might be beneficial?
- What else can we do to slow the progression of the disease?
- What happens if my loved one can't drive anymore; will you help us tell them?
- Does my loved one need any updated lab tests or medical imaging, such as an MRI? (This question is important if no imaging has been completed yet.)
- Will you provide documentation for FMLA (Family Medical Leave Act)? I am interested in pursuing this so I can be home to help my loved one.

Preparing for your office visit with your loved one will maximize the quality of your time with the doctor. Make it a priority to keep track of changes that your loved one is experiencing, and you'll be rewarded with accurate information and helpful feedback.

## SELF-CARE

As the disease progresses, you may need to implement some lifestyle changes of your own to help accommodate the changing world of both you and your loved one. You'll want to keep your life as balanced as possible, whatever that means for you. For some people, it may be time to think about cutting back on extra commitments and obligations that deplete your time and energy. Your life is different now. That can be a hard thing to accept, but in order to have energy and avoid burnout, you may need to prioritize and cut something from the list of activities so you have more time for the most important things in your life. Conversely, for others, it may be imperative to keep that extra commitment because it brings satisfaction and stress relief. The difference here is that you may need to prioritize that which rejuvenates your spirit and brings you joy, satisfaction, and companionship. If you're part of a book club, it may become too much; others may need that social connection. If you volunteer your time to help others, maybe it's time to step down for a while—after all, you're helping others in your personal life, too! Or maybe you thrive on that and wish to stay. Your sense of balance will dictate what works for you.

As the disease progresses, the demands placed upon you will increase. If you get depleted and worn out, this can lead to unnecessary crisis situations. So, take care of you. Even the simple things in life can be the most rewarding. Here are some ideas:

- Catch a nap.
- Cuddle with your pet.
- Watch your favorite movie.
- Find something to laugh about.
- Take a walk.
- Call or write an old friend.
- Exercise.
- Enjoy a cup of herbal tea.
- Jot down your thoughts in a journal.
- Keep moving throughout the day; stand and stretch often.

Self-care is a priority that will serve both you and your loved one well. Whatever helps to build you up, do it!

## JUST ONE THING

You are amazing, although some days you may not feel like it! On those days, do something nice for yourself. The smallest acts of kindness, even to oneself, can have a large impact on the human spirit. The kindness you show to your loved one must also be shown to yourself.

 Always say 'yes' to the present moment.... Surrender to what is.... Say 'yes' to life—and see how life starts suddenly to start working for you rather than against you."

—ECKHART TOLLE

CHAPTER FOUR

# An Alzheimer's Diagnosis

## JACKSON'S STORY

A retired automotive instructor, Jackson always needed to be busy, having no desire to sit still or slow down. He was always out in the yard, cutting and splitting firewood, mowing, raking, and never stopped moving all day long. His daughter, Juanita, realized that her dad had been having difficulty keeping up with the house for the past few years, and he was exhibiting some memory issues. Recently, Jackson injured himself while using a chainsaw. He needed more than 100 stitches, and the healing was taking longer than expected. In speaking with his doctor, Juanita asked if the accident could have been caused by Jackson's trouble with his memory. The doctor reassured Juanita that it was just an accident, but that Jackson should not cut wood in the future. Deep down, Juanita thought that this accident could have been prevented if he didn't heat with wood or use the chainsaw anymore. She also knew that he can be quite stubborn at times and that, when he sets his mind on something, he rarely changes it.

## What to Expect

For the caregiver, this time of diagnosis and realization can be complicated and challenging, but it is very necessary in order for you to understand what's to come. Your loved one may have had a diagnosis of Alzheimer's for some time, or perhaps they are just recently diagnosed. If this is your first experience with the reality of Alzheimer's, you will begin to learn to adapt to an ever-changing new normal. Issues that arise may include communication deficits, an increasing inability for your loved one to mask their confusion, and, often, the need to make decisions about retirement and new ways to spend time. We'll talk more about how life may change and what you might expect from your loved one. We'll also look at what you can do to help throughout these transitions, as you come to grips with this serious diagnosis.

## MILD-MODERATE COGNITIVE IMPAIRMENT

When an older adult develops problems with memory and thinking, very often it starts as mild cognitive impairment (also known as MCI). As the disease progresses, your loved one will develop increased difficulty with tasks and more frequent confusion and memory loss. Transitioning from mild to mild-moderate cognitive impairment presents new challenges for both the older adult and the caregiver. Generally, this is when the family and caregiver really notice the changes in their loved one, as it becomes increasingly difficult for the older adult to mask their memory loss and confusion. Complex tasks that were once manageable for them can become overwhelming, and diminished judgment may cause your loved one to make poor decisions. You may notice that their visual perception has gotten worse or that their driving skills have declined.

If your loved one is still working, their job may become difficult for them, and they may even be at risk for unemployment. Very often, this is when people make the decision to retire, either by choice or not. If your loved one is still working, it may be wise to have a conversation about exiting the workforce before the situation gets worse. The older adult may be fearful or embarrassed about their diminishing abilities. As the caregiver, supporting them as they make the difficult decision to leave their employment can be a great gift to protect their reputation and dignity. Conversely, it could also trigger your loved one to dig their heels in and refuse to retire. This defiance may be caused by the progression of the disease, as the older adult is unable to grasp what is really happening. Being stubborn and refusing to let go of something that is important to them can be part of the disease or just their natural personality. It's important to differentiate between what is caused by the progression of the disease, and what are normal personality traits that are exacerbated due to changes in your loved one's ability to manage their emotions.

Another factor that may influence their decision to retire is that your loved one's identity may be intricately linked to their role in the workforce. Perhaps they are a nurse, teacher, secretary, plumber, firefighter, cook, mechanic, etc. The thought of not being that person may be sad, even terrifying, for that older adult. Part of your role as caregiver can be to support your loved one as they face an increasingly profound identity crisis, due to the progression of the disease. The transition caused by the loss of a career can be devastating to your loved one, triggering grief and regret for all the things that will not be in the future. This can be nearly as devastating for the caregiver, as the situation can no longer be avoided or ignored.

## INSIDE ALZHEIMER'S

This stage, transitioning from the mild to the almost moderate stage of the disease, is a pivotal time. The older adult might be ashamed and embarrassed because they can no longer do some of the most important activities in their day-to-day life. Their brain is not functioning normally in some ways. However, the older adult may feel like they can still do many of the tasks that they once did without difficulty. For Jackson (see Jackson's Story, page 53), the task of cutting wood might be complicated by his inability to consider certain details. He may not realize that the chain needs to be sharpened and that the gas may need to be mixed with oil for proper functioning. Jackson may no longer understand that he needs to wear ear and eye protection when he cuts wood. It's pretty clear to everyone around him that Jackson can no longer cut wood, and so his daughter may need a plan to help Jackson transition to doing other tasks that are safe and manageable for him. Jackson may feel frustrated and angry and not understand why his daughter is after him to stop cutting wood. As a caregiver, this may be when you hear "I'm fine" 100 times, and you know that they're not!

# What to Say

As the disease progresses from the mild to the mild-moderate stages, the older adult will probably have a difficult time adapting to changing roles and understanding that they need additional support. These times of transition can be very stressful for everyone involved, but you can help by spinning things in a thoughtful and sensitive way. When referring to your loved one retiring, for example, it's important to acknowledge their successes and recognize that this is a very difficult time for them.

Surely, you can empathize with their situation—their life's passion may be drawing to a close! You'll want to be gentle in your approach. You can even help your loved one come to the decision on their own, sort of. You may need to be creative, saying, "You've worked your whole life, and now it's time to take a break, take it easy, and open a new chapter in life. Do you think there's something you might want to spend more time doing?"

If you find that the best approach is the direct one, you could further point out that, by retiring, they would avoid any damage being done, their reputation being tarnished, and the risk of being fired. One way to word this might be, "Dad, you've worked hard for a long time, and you have a good reputation. Better to exit the workplace on your terms and not someone else's." Or, "Mom, we are all worried about you—you've gotten lost on your way home from work. How can we help? We want to keep you safe."

As a caregiver, of course you'll want to protect your loved one from situations that can cause embarrassment or distress for them. But, when you're met with opposition from them, an interim compromise may be necessary as you continue to advocate for their safety and well-being.

As for Jackson, coming to a compromise about cutting wood may involve finding a new source of heat for his home. If he disagrees, Juanita could suggest moving as an alternative. She would be calling his bluff—most people want to stay in their home and will often agree to a compromise in order to remain there.

For caregivers, finding the right words can be one of the most stressful parts of being a caregiver. If this is a parent, your roles have switched from cared-for to caregiver, and this can be awkward. But it's the new reality. From this point on, you will be heading into areas that require difficult conversations from time to time. At this stage, your loved one still maintains much of their personality and preferences, and you most likely know their preferred communication style. As communication needs change with the progression of the disease, you'll continue to figure out how to navigate this complicated journey. To that end, I'll offer practical tips and suggestions to implement as you navigate the twists and turns that lie ahead.

## What to Do

During this transition, knowing what to do may be clear and obvious, or you may not have a clue where to begin. This is natural! Most likely, this is a new role for you, and the issues and needs are ever-changing. Just as every older adult experiences the progression of the disease differently, every caregiver experiences the journey differently, too. You may intuitively know what needs to be done, but how do you make it happen, keeping in mind your loved one's opinion and rights? Knowing what to do and executing it should be done with a mind toward best preserving their dignity, resources, and independence, and all of that must be done safely. Yes, it's complicated. But you don't need to go it alone.

Seek out help from family members who are good at problem solving and will have your back. Support groups can also be a wonderful resource, through which you can learn from other caregivers what they do in similar situations. Finally, don't forget to seek out assistance from your loved one's physician. They are a trusted and experienced ally to whom you can turn as your responsibilities increase.

## TAPPING INTO BENEFITS

A variety of programs are available that allow families to be paid to care for their loved one. These programs and their eligibility criteria vary by state. You can start by reaching out to your county and state offices for aging or senior services. Ask for information about consumer-directed or self-directed programs in your area. On the federal level, the Family Medical Leave Act has a provision for employees to take a leave of absence to provide care for a seriously ill spouse, child, or parent that ensures your job is protected. See Resources (page 160) for website links.

## FINDING THE RIGHT DOCTOR

In your quest to find the right doctor to diagnose and treat Alzheimer's, you may wish to start with your loved one's primary care provider (PCP). Many PCPs do a tremendous job in assessing and diagnosing Alzheimer's disease.

The Alzheimer's Association estimates that a skilled physician can diagnose Alzheimer's disease with more than 90 percent accuracy. To follow up on specific symptoms such as memory loss or thinking issues, you'll want to find a doctor that you and your loved one feel comfortable with. Most people initially contact their PCP or internist about their concerns regarding memory loss and trouble with thinking, and the PCP often is at the center of the diagnostic process. If the PCP has not assessed your loved one for memory loss, or dismisses your concerns, or if your loved one's symptoms become difficult to manage, it may be advantageous to see a specialist.

A neurologist specializes in diseases of the brain and nervous system. Many neurologists are very capable of getting an accurate diagnosis, and they can provide support with medication management and dealing with difficult behaviors and other symptoms throughout the progression of the disease.

A geriatrician specializes in the care of older adults. This specialist can provide an accurate diagnosis of Alzheimer's disease, based on their experience working with older adults.

Finding the right doctor can make all the difference in getting an accurate diagnosis and ongoing support. Ideally, seek a physician who makes you and your loved one feel valued and comfortable when asking questions—this partnership will allow for the lines of communication to be open, and, with luck, this professional will be an integral part of your team for the duration.

If your questions aren't being answered to your satisfaction, don't give up. Give the current physician a few more calls, and demand to have your questions addressed. Don't be dismissed—your loved one needs an accurate diagnosis. If this was a medical condition such as cancer, cardiac disease, or a bowel-related illness, you would absolutely receive a diagnosis, probably with a prognosis, as well. Alzheimer's disease is a medical condition that will benefit from proper treatment and support to help manage symptoms and complications as the disease progresses. If you are not satisfied, seek out a second opinion! Every caregiver and patient needs accurate information; that's why it's so important to partner with a physician who will listen to you or who has staff who are willing and able to do so. Be persistent and brave in your quest to build a team whose members are available to help and will listen when you call. Caregiver support and education groups can also offer encouragement and be very empowering when difficult topics need to be addressed.

## PLANNING AHEAD

As you're learning about Alzheimer's disease—the stages and symptoms, finding the right doctor, tracking down a diagnosis, and beginning this journey of caregiving—there are a few more important details that are best addressed sooner rather than later. As your loved one's memory and thinking abilities are at risk of declining, now is the time to start the conversation about planning for the future. In the early stages of the disease, the older adult still has the ability to make decisions about their future. How and where they will live in this next chapter of their life is something they will want to consider. Also, who might they wish to designate to help make decisions about health care, legal, and financial matters? Creating a living will and identifying a power of attorney and health care proxy are essential tasks that should be addressed in the early stages. A living will provides information about the type of care that your loved one wishes and documents the type of care allowed when your loved one lacks capacity or is no longer able to speak for themself. A health care proxy (HCP) is a person designated by the older adult, who is available to make medical decisions if the older adult

## WHAT TO ASK THE DOCTOR

As I will continue to stress, when you visit the doctor, grab your notebook with all your wonderful, detailed notes. One of the best things you can do is prepare for the visit by writing down your observations, questions, and concerns beforehand. It sounds so simple, but it is positively critical to getting your loved one an accurate diagnosis and the treatment and care they deserve. Whatever you do, please do not send your loved one alone. The physician will need your input. You will provide valuable information that is essential in making an accurate diagnosis. You also want to be present to make sure everything is being explained clearly and honestly and that the doctor's feedback is fully understood.

You can refer to your notes and explain:

- What's going on?
- When did it start?
- How long it has been going on?

You may want to ask the following questions:

- Will my loved one's memory be assessed or tested?
- What tests will they do, what does the testing involve, and will these tests be given at future visits? (This will assist in tracking changes over time.)

is unable to speak for themselves. In the early stages, your loved one can be very active in making their healthcare decisions. As the disease progresses, the HCP will be responsible for making sure that your loved one's wishes are carried out. The HCP must be available to speak on behalf of your loved one. They must be part of the planning discussions with the loved one, so they know what their wishes and choices are. The HCP can be the primary caregiver or not; the decision is made by your loved one.

The power of attorney (POA) is another very important role that gives a designated person authority to make financial decisions on

- How long will the appointment take?
- When will we learn the results?
- Does the physician need any other documentation, such as recent lab results from other physicians?

When you go to the appointment, you will always want to bring a list of current medications, including over-the-counter medications, vitamins, and supplements, as well as their dosages.

If your loved one has had medical imaging, you will want to bring a digital or hard copy or make sure that the physician gets the image in advance. Medical imaging can be ordered by the PCP, neurologist, or another authorized healthcare professional. These include MRIs or CT scans, which are pictures and images of the brain that can be used to help diagnose Alzheimer's disease.

One more factor to consider when talking with your doctor: It can be upsetting for all when you're listing the deficits and problems that are occurring with your loved one's memory and thinking abilities. Printing or writing a list and handing it to the nurse is respectful and discreet and can help to avoid emotional responses. You may even request to speak with the nurse or other appropriate staff person privately to express your concerns.

behalf of the loved one. This is memorialized by a legal document that, ideally, should be completed with the help of an attorney. If that is cost-prohibitive, as not everyone can afford a lawyer, these can be completed in most states by the loved one and the designated person. The document needs to be notarized by an authorized notary public. Most banks and county offices have notaries on staff.

Be very selective about who is chosen to be the POA. This individual legally has access to any money and resources that are in the name of your loved one. This person must be honest and ethical. It's also important to be sure that the form is completed properly; if not, the POA could be voided. As the disease progresses, the POA allows the designated person to pay the bills and spend money on care for the loved one. A trusted POA will help ease some of the caregiving burden by managing the financial aspect of your loved one's life.

Getting these plans underway can be very stressful for the caregiver! Opinions and personal agendas can create turmoil in the family, especially when starting these conversations and talking about sensitive issues. It may not be an easy task to get such affairs in order, but it's crucial. It may take multiple attempts to make progress and come to agreements with these matters, as well as time to complete documents. This time spent facing the reality of the disease can be devastating for everyone. It can be helpful to hire an attorney and to consult your loved one's physician, who can provide trusted guidance for your loved one, and whose presence may reduce the chance that family turmoil will erupt.

## CAREGIVING: PLANNING AHEAD

In an ideal world, plans for the future would be in place, healthcare wishes would be fully understood, a trustworthy POA would be designated, everyone would be in agreement, and your loved one would be completely on board with all of this. That is a beautiful scenario, but most likely it's not realistic. In the journey ahead, there will be twists and turns, unanticipated delays, and unplanned detours. That said, take some time in the early stages to learn about the available services and resources that you may need as time goes on. This is the time to seek out information so you're prepared when the need arises.

Here are a few common topics you may want to learn more about:

- If your older adult is a veteran, their service is valued and appreciated! Take some time now to learn about available benefits connected to their service. Not every veteran is eligible for support services, but many are. As their health status changes and the disease progresses, there may be additional support services available to help meet their changing needs.
- Look into services such as free legal clinics, home health agencies that provide care, and volunteer outreach programs that provide companionship for loved ones. There are also programs that pay for a family member to provide caregiver services (see page 160). These vary from state to state and have eligibility criteria.
- Learn all you can about your loved one's insurance, if any benefits or support services are available, and the associated eligibility requirements that may be needed to access services. It may be easier to call their health insurance company and speak to a human than to try to glean information from a thick packet of insurance documentation.
- Explore various organizations. Does your county or state office for aging have programs? If you need help finding adaptive equipment, such as a walker or shower chair, who provides that? Can you find a free geriatric care manager or care navigator through the Alzheimer's Association or office for aging? On the Internet, search "services for older adults with Alzheimer's disease near me" and see what pops up. Or, search "caregiver support services near me." These general search terms will help give you direction as to what's available in your area. Don't be afraid to make phone calls and ask questions. Even if you don't find the right information or people immediately, you'll eventually get pointed in the right direction.
- Ask questions, and partner with all of your loved one's health care team members. Ask the nurse, social worker, and doctor if they can direct you to support services for help. If the doctor recommends that your loved one get some socialization, ask them how to make that happen. Get in the habit of asking questions when a suggestion is made. When recommendations are made, write down their suggestions in your notebook, which hopefully, you have grown quite attached to.

- Explore the differences between Medicare and Medicaid, and learn who provides what services. Most caregivers scramble to learn about services right when they're needed—either in the heat of the crisis or shortly thereafter. Why not know all of this going in? Knowing the difference between these insurance providers will be helpful. Medicare does not pay for long-term care but will pay for short-term rehabilitation services. Medicaid will provide more care and is the insurance coverage for people with lower incomes. There are many nuances to Medicare and Medicaid and other insurances. In many communities, seminars are available to help learn the ins and outs of these services. Many county offices for aging have insurance specialists available to answer questions.
- Learn who may not be helpful at all at this point. There are service providers who do not serve older adults, due to age restrictions. There may be an adult day program that serves only visually impaired people. Or, there may be geriatric care managers available that charge for services. Other programs base eligibility on income. If your loved one's income exceeds a certain threshold, they will not be able to access those services. But, again, don't be afraid to ask questions: Do they make exceptions to those guidelines? If your loved one has vast medical expenses, can that be a contributing factor to determine eligibility? Ask about exceptions and explain your needs—you might get surprising results. This is the time to determine who is on your team, to avoid scrambling later.

## Self-Care

In these early stages of the journey, self-care may feel like an unnecessary need for the caregiver. However, now is the time to build your support network, knowing that your needs will continue to evolve as the disease progresses and the needs of your loved one change. Taking care of yourself is a concept and habit that should be firmly rooted in these early stages. When your loved one knows that you'll be there for them, but that you'll also be taking care of yourself, this will set a clear expectation that being healthy is a priority that will benefit both of you.

It's valuable to know ahead of time where to turn for support as you face this disease and watch your loved one change over time. A support group is a good place to get solidarity and emotional guidance from others in similar situations. As we've explored already, making self-care a priority is perhaps one of the most important decisions you'll make to positively impact your health and wellness, especially as you watch someone you care about decline over time. Getting exercise, eating healthy food, doing something that you love (other than caregiving), and getting enough sleep can make profound differences in how well you manage the stress of caregiving.

## SELF-COMPASSION

You probably never thought that you'd be a caregiver at this point in your life. The realization of caregiving can be overwhelming, rewarding, and HARD. You are doing the best you can; you are ethical, honest, loving, and very special. You may not agree with those statements today, but please know that there is no greater gift that you can give on this planet than to do the very best you can for yourself when your loved one has Alzheimer's disease. Take care of yourself and give yourself a break—the same break that you would grant to others.

### JUST ONE THING

You as the caregiver are facing a complicated journey ahead. Take a moment and think about just one thing that you could do for yourself today—something small that could have a powerful, positive impact on your attitude and point of view. These are the moments that will help you take a break and catch your breath in a time when most of the focus is on someone else. No matter how quick the moment, take it, enjoy it, and do it again, each and every day.

 Talk to yourself like you would to someone you love."

—BRENÉ BROWN

# CHAPTER FIVE

# At Home

## BOBBI'S STORY

Sara and Bobbi had been devoted to each other for over 20 years. They traveled the world and were ready to experience their next adventure together. They loved to hike and experience different cultures. Sara recently retired from the corporate world, while Bobbi had stopped working several years ago, after 30 years as a pediatric nurse in a hospital. She loved children and was kind and gentle with them. When Bobbi started to have problems with her memory, she decided that it was time to retire. Actually, Bobbi had been making some mistakes on the job and was finally encouraged by her coworkers and Sara to retire. She retired with her benefits and reputation intact. Shortly after her retirement, Bobbi was diagnosed with Alzheimer's disease. Sara and Bobbi enjoyed several more years doing things together, until Bobbi could no longer travel. She now needs someone to be near her all the time to make sure that she stays safe. Thankfully, Bobbi is generally good-natured and agreeable to Sara's suggestions.

## What to Expect

Now that your loved one has entered the moderate stage of the disease, a safe and comfortable home is one of the most important things you can provide for them. A familiar place with all the things that make their house a home—the sounds, the sights, the smells—are essential to feeling secure. Your loved one may still know the comfort of their favorite chair or blanket. And, of course, pets can provide an enormous amount of comfort and pleasure. Familiar places and people can be very reassuring for your loved one, even as their memory fades. When they have trouble remembering and thinking, they still need your reassurance and the comfort of those things that were once familiar to them. As the disease progresses, changes will impact your loved one's ability to do many of the things that they've done their entire life. For example, your loved one has made coffee for 50 years, but recently they turned on the coffee pot and didn't add water, so the coffee pot burned and broke. Your loved one has had a muffin for breakfast every day, warmed up in the microwave— but now they don't remember which buttons to push.

Generally, by this stage, your loved one is still quite capable of eating and drinking, but assembling the food and drinks becomes increasingly challenging. All the steps involved in getting a plate, glass, fork, and napkin, putting the food on the plate, heating it up, carrying it to the table, and pouring a drink can be very complicated for your loved one. Therefore, it's important for you as the caregiver to be sure that your loved one is eating and drinking enough every day. Getting enough water is absolutely essential—remind them to drink and take frequent sips of water. Dehydration is a common reason that older adults end up in the emergency room with increased confusion, injuries from falls, and urinary tract infections. Make it a habit and your mission to be the "water police," and offer water throughout the day, every day.

## FALL RISKS

Your loved one may not yet have many physical limitations caused by the disease. However, over time, as the disease progresses, the brain plays tricks on the eyes, and as such, your loved one may develop difficulty interpreting the things that they are seeing. This creates an increased risk for falls and trips. For example, your loved one may put on shoes that are too large or forget to use their walker, or they may have trouble with balance, all of which create a risk for falls. Alzheimer's disease interferes with how the brain interprets what your loved one is seeing. It can also alter their depth perception. They may miscalculate where the step is, causing them to trip and fall. You may notice that they are holding onto the stair railing very tightly or grasping your arm, depending on you to help them navigate the stairs. Offer gentle reassurance, and make a note in your notebook that this is a new challenge your loved one is having.

## EXTERNAL DISTRACTIONS

Your loved one may develop new sensitivities to noises or shadows during the day. It's also common for an older adult to feel uncomfortable with new people coming into the home. Even a person who was once very social may no longer want to meet new people or be around groups of people. This can prove a challenge for the caregiver when they need to bring someone into the home. The caregiver will need to get creative in explaining why the person is in the home. If possible, recruit people to help who know your loved one and will be comfortable if the situation gets a little tense. You can ease the transition by orienting this person to the needs of your loved one. Some older adults will never agree to have someone come into the home in place of the primary caregiver. In those situations, other family members may need to step up and help out when possible.

As a caregiver, making sure that your loved one's home is safe and secure will be one of the most important tasks you'll need to accomplish. Don't worry about doing this all at once. Just as the disease progresses gradually, so will the necessity to secure the home. Take notice of your loved one's changing abilities and needs, and recognize that they will continue to change and you'll need to adjust for that as time goes on.

For example, when Bobbi (see Bobbi's Story, page 67) first retired, Sara could leave her at home alone for several hours. As the disease progressed, however, Sara realized that she could no longer leave Bobbi home alone. Bobbi had left the stove burner on and had no recollection of using the stove at all. Another time, Bobbi was going to wash the dishes, but she became distracted and walked away from the sink—the water overflowed all over the kitchen floor. Fortunately, Sara was home for that one and discovered the overflow before any serious damage was done. As safety is paramount, adapting the home to keep your loved one safe is the highest priority and, ultimately, the most important part of being the caregiver for a loved one who has Alzheimer's disease.

## INSIDE ALZHEIMER'S

In the moderate stage of Alzheimer's disease, the brain continues to shrink, and processing information becomes increasingly hard. Take a moment and try to put yourself in the shoes of your loved one. Imagine that you need to go to the grocery store. When you put your glasses on to look at your shopping list, the left lens of your glasses is foggy, and, in the background, you hear constant static—not very loud, but enough to interfere with your concentration. You put on your shoes, and the right foot feels tight, but you're not sure why. You can't seem to find your wallet; you look and look for it, but you just don't know where it is. Gasp, maybe someone came in and stole it—that's it, someone took your wallet! You're really upset now. You empty out all the drawers in the desk and still can't find it.

This is a moment-to-moment, daily occurrence for a person with Alzheimer's. What's actually happening is that your loved one is having problems processing and managing all the steps that are needed to go grocery shopping. They are hearing phantom noises and are suspicious because their brain isn't functioning properly. You discover that the wallet is in the washer, and they have emptied out their dresser drawers, not the desk. There are clothes on the floor, and your loved one is anxious and upset. The noises that they are hearing are actually coming from the TV.

Taking an occasional glimpse into your loved one's experience will help you be extra patient and gentle in your responses to the unique situations that you encounter. Remember, to your loved one, it all makes perfect sense.

## What to Say

During the moderate stage of Alzheimer's disease, adjustments will need to be made in most or all areas of your loved one's life. Communication can become tricky as your loved one has increased difficulty processing all that you're saying to them. Try to keep your questions, requests, and statements short and simple. You can help them feel reassured by talking in a calm voice, especially when they're feeling overwhelmed and confused. For example, when Sara discovered water pouring all over the kitchen floor, Bobbi was standing there, looking out the window and asking, "Where's Rascal?" Sara was furious. She wanted to scream at Bobbi and ask, "What's wrong with you? Don't you see the water all over the floor? And our dog died last year!" Instead, Sara took a deep breath and said, "Bobbi, come into the living room while I clean up the mess in the kitchen. We'll look for Rascal in a little while."

Sara cleaned up the mess with tears streaming down her face, as she watched her partner deteriorate before her eyes. But she knew that when she was calm, Bobbi was easier to manage and stayed calm as well. This happened last week—Sara did yell at Bobbi, and Bobbi began crying hysterically and apologized repeatedly. Then Bobbi didn't sleep at all that night because she knew that she did something that made Sara upset. Being calm and kind in the midst of difficult situations is hard but beneficial for everyone involved. When we blow up, it depletes our energy, and you know you really need that energy!

While we're talking about saving energy, consider this one: If and when your loved one becomes fixated on a topic, repeating the same question over and over again, you don't necessarily have to give them the full explanation every time they ask the question. They may ask, "When is the appointment?" and then repeat that question 30 times before you go. It's okay to reply, "In a little while" or "At noon," even if the appointment is tomorrow or next week. Just use your judgment and tell them whatever it takes to keep everyone calm.

When an appointment is scheduled, you may want to wait to tell them until just before it's time to go. This can help minimize your loved one's uncertainty and the repetition of the same question in the week preceding the appointment. As the disease progresses, it manifests itself in fears about having to leave the home or being separated from you. Therefore, when it comes to communication, sometimes the less said, the better.

# What to Do

The need to adapt and be flexible is another great challenges of caring for someone with Alzheimer's disease. Changes will occur that interfere with well-established routines; as you go, consider these practical tips and strategies for keeping everyone safe:

- If using the stove has become a danger, take the knobs off the stove and hide them. If your loved one is still living alone, you can disable the stove by turning off the power source and unplugging it.
- If your loved one can still make coffee, a coffee maker with an automatic shutoff can be very helpful.
- Use automatic timers to turn lights or other items on and off at appropriate times.
- Make sure the carbon monoxide and smoke detectors are in working order. Many local fire departments can assist with that task.
- Remove small appliances that may become dangerous if they are not operated properly. Sharp knives should also be removed to prevent your loved one from injuring themselves.
- If there is a garbage disposal in the sink, it should be disengaged to prevent your loved one from breaking it or hurting themself by putting in foreign objects.
- Look around with a critical eye. For example, if they have magnets on the refrigerator that look like fruit or food, you'll want to remove them when your loved one has increased confusion, as they could mistake them for food.
- Put lock boxes over the thermostat. This will prevent them from making radical changes to the heat or air conditioning.
- Add a new lock to the basement door when it's no longer be safe for them to go down the stairs or to be alone around the furnace, hot water heater, or electrical box. Put the lock up at the top of the door, out of sight, to deter them.
- Remove axes, chainsaws, and other power tools.
- Keep chemicals out of reach, such as bleach, bathroom disinfectants, and other products that could be dangerous.

As you now well know, Alzheimer's disease impairs a person's judgment and ability to make safe choices. When you remove the dangerous items, it removes the temptation, keeping your loved one safe and arguments and fights at bay.

It's okay to ask for help in some of these areas. Get a team together, and put all of the safety measures in place that you can. By adapting the home and keeping your loved one safe, you will enable them to live safely and independently for as long as possible. As the level of dependence increases, safety is a growing priority. By adapting the home and environment, you will enable your loved to safely age in place.

Once you've created the safest possible living space, you can learn to enjoy the moments that you share with your loved one. Even as they descend further into the moderate stage, there are moments of joy and fun that can be carved out—look for them! Try to be present and mindful in the moment with your loved one. These moments are gifts. In the case of Sara and Bobbi, after Sara cleaned up the mess on the kitchen floor, they went and sat on the porch. Their cat jumped on Bobbi's lap. Bobbi smiled and started to lovingly stroke the cat, and then she suddenly started singing her favorite song, "Rock with You," by Michael Jackson. Together they sang the song imperfectly, holding hands and appreciating a rare moment in time when they were once again partners. Together, they laughed when the cat covered her ears with her paws as they sang.

Join your loved one for a moment when they tell a story about their life—you may have heard it a thousand times, but just relax and try to enjoy their company in that moment. Even though they have Alzheimer's disease, they may still have moments of clarity, laughter, and love. Pull out some photos and reminisce; they may not recognize everyone in each photo, but they'll feel that sense of connectedness. Or, they might surprise you and remember more than you expected, prompted by the visual cues. Appreciate a positive moment that you can share with your loved one. As the great mid-century comedian Victor Borge said, "Laughter is the shortest distance between two people." The dishes can wait—go ahead and enjoy these moments with your loved one.

## WHAT TO ASK THE DOCTOR

As the moderate stage progresses, your relationship with the doctor is very important. By now, if you aren't satisfied with the care and attention that your loved one is receiving, be brave and seek out a second opinion. Your loved one's quality of life is so important. It can take years for your loved one to move through the moderate stage of the disease. This is a good time to make modifications that will allow your loved one to stay at home. Ask the physician:

- What can we expect over the next several months or year?
- How long will my loved one be in the moderate stage?
- Is there a way to slow the progression of the disease?
- Does Alzheimer's run in the family? As a family member, is there anything I can do to reduce my chances of getting it?
- Are there any supplements that may be beneficial at this stage?

# Self-Care

Making time for self-care may be challenging at times. You may even need some extra incentive. For example, if you really need a break, how about planning something really special for yourself to look forward to? It doesn't need to be expensive or extravagant. Think about answering, "I could really go for a _____". As long as it's legal, plan it! Could you really go for a nice meal out, a picnic on a blanket, meeting up with your friend? Take your favorite little person, perhaps a grandchild, to the park for some fun. How about curling up with a book? Maybe watch a TV show or listen to a podcast that will nourish your spirit or make you laugh or inspire you to appreciate yourself and the precious gifts that you are giving your loved one. TED Talks provide thousands of short lectures on hundreds of different topics. These talks are inspiring, funny, and thought-provoking. Many are quite short; some are only about three minutes long and provide a quick respite when you really need one (see Resources, page 160).

Your self-care doesn't need to be complicated; keep it simple if that's all you can manage right now. Plan something special and take some time to enjoy the moment. It will be time well spent, an investment in your health and wellness.

As you keep your loved one safe at home, it's imperative that you take care of yourself. It's important not to lose your identity on this journey. Regularly try to do something for yourself that is apart from your loved one.

## JUST ONE THING

Let's set the record straight: You're definitely not the bad guy. But, you're making tough decisions that may initially upset your loved one. They may lash out or take out their frustration and fear on you. You may be unpopular from time to time, because your loved one does not understand why you're doing or saying certain things. Even others in the family may not understand why, for example, you're adapting the home environment. You're perhaps singlehandedly maintaining the dignity and quality of life of your loved one, and it can be overwhelming. When family members question you and become critical, this can really hurt! Know in your heart and soul that you're doing what is best for your loved one. If your family is being obstinate, invite them to take your loved one out for the afternoon or spend a weekend with them, and then maybe they'll have a better understanding. If they decide not to be helpful, let it go as best as you can, and move on. Your time and energy are precious and cannot be wasted on someone who will not be helpful. This is why your self-care is so important. Try to focus on the rewards of being a caregiver. There's no greater gifts you can give your loved one than the ones you are already giving—treating them with dignity and respect and keeping them safe. Now, give yourself a gift by treating yourself with love, kindness, and encouragement.

 Every single person is sacred. Sacred means special, precious, a treasure of true beauty. That means you."

—AMY LEIGH MERCREE

# CHAPTER SIX

# Out in the World

## RUSSELL'S STORY

Russell is a proud veteran. He was awarded the Silver Star for his bravery while serving his country in the Vietnam War. As a career soldier, Russell came back to the United States after his tour of duty and was stationed at several different military bases. He married his high school sweetheart, Lenore, just before he was drafted, and together they had three children. Lenore and the kids lived on four different bases while Russell traveled, and when the kids were in high school, Lenore and Russell decided not to move again until all the kids had graduated. Lenore was then diagnosed with breast cancer, and Russell requested a transfer to be closer to home to help care for his sick wife. Lenore passed away at the age of 40. Russell decided to retire from the service to take care of his teenage children. He devoted his life to the kids, making sure that they all graduated and went to college, the workforce, or the military.

The years have passed, and now Russell has been diagnosed with moderate-stage Alzheimer's disease. Russell's children adore their dad and are committed to helping him to stay safely at home with his independence and dignity. Two of them live nearby, and they'll provide as much support as needed. Russell is kind but stern—he adheres to a strict routine, a result of having served in the military for over 30 years. The progression of Alzheimer's disease has been devastating for Russell. The loss of control that this career serviceman is facing has tipped his world upside down.

# What to Expect

As the disease progresses, changes will take place in your loved one's ability to navigate the world outside of the home. Familiar routines and places may become increasingly difficult to manage. This part of the journey will require you to be flexible and patient, as merely getting out of the house can involve the need for patience and creativity, and the changes happening are now being recognized by people outside of the home.

## PUBLIC OUTBURSTS

Even though every person experiences the progression of Alzheimer's disease differently, there is one common experience that caregivers generally share. This is when people outside of the family start to recognize that something is "just not right" with your loved one. This is a very important shift for caregivers, as they are now facing this disease in public spaces, outside the privacy of the home.

When your loved one is out in public and has an angry outburst or starts to say things that don't make any sense, the best solution is to go with the flow. The goal here is to keep your loved one and yourself calm in the midst of an embarrassing event. Perhaps your loved one is frustrated and they slam their fist on the table at the restaurant and start yelling at you. Or they throw their hands up in the air and walk out. This may trigger wandering, as the person with the disease is trying to leave an uncomfortable situation. (We'll discuss that more shortly.)

Your loved one may start to make inappropriate remarks that could have a sexual or otherwise inappropriate connotation. Some people with Alzheimer's disease lose the ability to process the thoughts that pop into their heads, and are no longer able to filter those thoughts to determine what is appropriate to be said out loud. For example, if your loved one calls someone old or fat or ugly, this can be embarrassing for everyone in close proximity. If this is something that your loved one has always done, then it's not Alzheimer's disease; it's normal behavior for that person.

However, very often, your loved one will be able to manage their actions when they are around other people. This is especially true when they have you there to guide the interactions and cover for them. However, when Alzheimer's disease interferes with your loved one's judgment, they may not comply or agree to things, such as going to an appointment. Your loved one might refuse to get in or out of the car at the appointment. As the caregiver, this is a good time to look around and evaluate who may be able to assist.

In Russell's case (see Russell's Story, page 77), as the disease progressed, his kids did not want him to stay at home alone all day. He attended an adult day program at the Veterans Administration Hospital, where he enjoyed socializing and being around other veterans. However, one day, Russell refused to get out of the car at the program. His son had to get to work, so it quickly escalated into a stressful situation. Russell said, "I'm not going there . . . [gibberish] . . . no!" The program staff saw that Russell was having a problem. They were able to intervene and get Russell into a wheelchair. His son took him to urgent care, and they discovered that Russell was dehydrated and had a lung infection. He recovered from that acute illness, but it triggered an unpleasant association for Russell each time he arrived at the day program. He became agitated and angry whenever they pulled up in front of the building. After much discussion and brainstorming, the staff allowed Russell to enter the program through the back door. With this creative intervention, Russell was able to attend the program for another year.

## MULTIPLE DOCTORS

As the disease progresses, your loved one may need to see more than one physician, and they may also experience other acute illnesses. Getting them to the doctor's office may require some creative action. Early on in the moderate stage, offering to stop for coffee, lunch, or ice cream can help motivate your loved one to go to the appointment. You may discover that if you delay telling your loved one about the appointment, it reduces anxiety. For your loved one, seeing a doctor may be scary and overwhelming, especially when it is a new doctor. Your loved one may still understand that physicians sometimes must give bad news to their patients. While this may not necessarily be true in your case, it may be helpful to wait to tell your loved one that you're going to an appointment until after they are on their way. It's a matter of being sensitive in making the effort to reduce feelings of anxiety or worry. This may not work for everyone, nor may it be necessary; some people love their doctor and will go to the appointment without hesitation.

## GETTING DRESSED AND BATHING

Your loved one may not want to change their clothes. It's very common for people with Alzheimer's disease to wear the same clothes over and over again. With the loss of functioning, there's also a loss of understanding about things like the importance of putting on clean clothes or even bathing. Both of these situations can be embarrassing and stressful for caregivers, and can quickly lead to epic battles, causing an enormous amount of stress and strain for everyone involved. One solution is to buy duplicate sets of clothes, and when they do take the outfit off, you can give them the fresh identical clothes to put on. Getting your loved one to change clothes and bathe may require time, patience, and, again, creativity. You can try telling them that the doctor wants them to put this shirt on and not to wear soiled pants. Think about who could be the "good guy" or the "bad guy" to help motivate your loved one. Blame the dog, the cat—whatever sparks that moment of compliance by your loved one.

There is another intervention that's proven successful and often used in skilled care facilities and nursing homes—singing! Yes, sing while you help your loved one change their clothes. Put on their favorite music and sing along. Of course, you may not feel like singing every time you need your loved one to change their clothes, bathe, or wash up. In fact, the last thing may you feel like doing is singing and being upbeat when you're making sure that your loved one bathes and puts on clean undergarments. This is where perspective comes in. Maybe it's time to bend the rules a bit and define a new normal. That may include having your loved one wear the same clothes (switching duplicate outfits) and just washing up as opposed to having a shower every day. Bathing a few times each week and washing up in between may become the new norm.

## DIGNITY AND AUTONOMY

Being flexible is vital to helping someone maintain their dignity and quality of life, while still making some of these tasks manageable for you. Part of the complexity of being a caregiver for someone with Alzheimer's disease lies in helping them maintain some degree of autonomy—for their good and for yours. It may not look so perfect on some days; in fact, depending on the day or the personality of your loved one and the trajectory of the disease, the current state of affairs will ultimately determine when and where you are able to take your loved one outside of the home. This will most likely change over time and perhaps frequently. Being flexible and patient can help you avoid and diffuse stressful situations.

As socializing becomes more challenging for your loved one, you'll discover who will be kind and understanding when interacting with them, and when it's safe to disclose the diagnosis. You may also develop a new set of skills that help protect your loved one in social situations. Protecting their dignity while keeping them safe is a precious gift. And yes, it can be exhausting for the caregiver to balance all of this! Take time to identify who your loved one will be safe and comfortable with as the disease progresses, and who will be there to help you along this journey. Build your tribe of supportive people—this can really make all the difference in the quality of your life and that of your loved one.

## INSIDE ALZHEIMER'S DISEASE

Your loved one is having more difficulty navigating the world and is needing more support. Take a moment and think about how you would act and feel if you broke your leg and were stuck in a cast up to your hip. Now, today, you need to go to a doctor's appointment, you aren't feeling well at all, you've had surgery, and you're still a little groggy and unfocused from the anesthesia. Your adult daughter tells you to change your clothes and wash up and be ready to go by noon. You're getting cold and don't know how you're going to get into the shower and get cleaned up. You can't get into your closet to get clean clothes and have no desire to wash your face or brush your teeth. Your leg is throbbing, and your opposite hip is sore from lying on it so much. Your daughter comes in and yells at you, "Why haven't you changed your clothes?" Now, suddenly, you're having a reaction to the pain medication and feel sick to your stomach. You're freezing cold, and you feel awful. You tell your daughter to cancel the appointment—you're staying home. She gets totally irate and tells you to change your clothes now and that you ARE going! You're overwhelmed, miserable, and not going anywhere!

For a moment, feel what your loved one may be experiencing. Don't focus on the pain of being in a cast; rather, think about not being able to get into the bathroom or reach your clothes, and feeling generally terrible. Think about having no desire to leave your home and feeling totally overwhelmed. As changes in the brain continue to develop, your loved one may feel safe and secure at home, and going out can be paralyzing to them. This is when an established routine, complete with flexible rules, can come in handy. They may not realize it at the time, but, ultimately, getting out of the house can be beneficial for both you and your loved one.

# What to Say

Communication at this stage may test your patience over and over again. Just know that helping your loved one change clothes, go to an event outside of the home, or attend an appointment *can* be accomplished. Enlist all the usual tools here: Speak slowly, keep it simple and direct, and offer visual cues to help convey your words. Maintain eye contact, and smile when appropriate.

Here are additional strategies for effective communication:

- Be creative by using the names of people that are important to your loved one. Even if they may not remember them, recalling a familiar name may trigger a positive response and foster cooperation. For example, you might say, "Mom (or Dad or _____) wants you to put these pants on" or "We need to make sure that you look good for _____" or "You wouldn't want _____ to see you in that wrinkled shirt."
- If you're eating out, you can pull the server aside and quietly explain, "My dad has a little trouble with his memory; please be patient with us."
- To encourage them to go out, use statements like, "Mom, Dr. Jones wants to see how well you're doing; let's go show her," or "Mom, your friends want to meet you for lunch today" (this may help get them to their adult day program or senior center).
- To explain why they can't use certain things, you can say, "Dad, the chainsaw broke; the chain fell off" or "The basement door is broken and we'll have to get it fixed soon."
- If they act out in the faith community, talk to the leader and explain the situation. If it becomes too overwhelming to attend, see if any members from the community will make a home visit or take your loved one out for coffee.
- When your family is asking about your loved one, be honest, but always with respect for their dignity. "Mom has Alzheimer's disease; the doctor said that she's in the middle stage right now.

We need to make sure she feels loved, safe, and comfortable. When you're with her, just be super patient and don't ask her for anything right now." And, of course, another valuable line: "I could use your help with this situation."

- Be patient. If you're out together and your loved one gets anxious, it's okay. Just leave the situation and reassure them that they are safe and loved, saying, "Not to worry, we're heading home."

## What to Do

Don't be afraid to face these challenges; in fact, be fearless and honest when you need to be. If you and your loved one go for coffee every morning, and now you see that they're having difficulty finding the cream and sugar, add it for them ahead of time, then hand the cup to your loved one. If you know and trust an employee at the café, you can say that your loved one is not feeling well and may need some help sometimes. You may decide not to share the diagnosis in order to protect them from others who may not be trustworthy. Continue to take your loved one out; if a situation becomes uncomfortable for either of you, simply get up, leave, and go home. As the disease progresses, you may find that one or both of you become increasingly isolated. It's more important than ever to stay connected to friends and family members and be part of a community where you'll both get support and compassion from people who care about you and your loved one. Be brave, and make the best of this part of the journey by refusing to be isolated.

## Self-Care

Taking your loved one out of the house can become a big undertaking, and when they don't want to change their clothes, it can be even tougher. Pick your battles! This will preserve your energy. If you haven't already, let go of making everything perfect, and get ready to adopt a new norm. Try to keep your sense of humor, and don't let what others say bother you. Be gentle with yourself—you're undoubtedly giving

## WHAT TO ASK THE DOCTOR

Make a list of your observations and questions, and be ready to discuss any changes that have occurred since the last visit, such as new behaviors and changes in behavior. Bring a list of all current medications and supplements and their dosages. Good questions to ask at this appointment may include:

- Is medication available to help manage anxiety or other symptoms? Are alternative treatments available to help that do not include medication (non-pharmacological)?
- What stage of Alzheimer's are they in?
- Are any medical tests needed or suggested at this time?
- What can we expect as the disease progresses?
- How much should my loved one be eating and drinking?
- Will they have trouble swallowing?
- What can I give Dad for constipation or diarrhea?
- What if they only want to eat sweets? Can I let them have two cookies after they have a few bites of something healthy?

far more than you're receiving. Maintaining your health and wellness is more important than ever. This part of the journey will most likely last a while. Your self-care is a priority, so don't fall into the habit of putting yourself second or on the back burner. Make time to have some fun. Don't let yourself get isolated or shut people out. If a family member doesn't understand, let it go! You're positively amazing on this challenging journey. Going with the flow, as they say, will help you let go of some of the unnecessary stress that can interfere with your health and wellness. Try for a moment to accept the fact that you are giving your loved one the most precious gift of all. When you're tired, you're entitled to take a break. Smile and accept some help when it becomes available. And take that time just for you, whether you go out dancing or just curl up and take a nap.

## JUST ONE THING

Each and every day, do just one thing for yourself. Something small. Then, take it a step further and keep a list of all the little, tiny things you do for yourself each day. Reflecting on the little things you do just for you will help you smile and be at peace with all of the good that you're doing. You may even find yourself looking forward to that one small thing!

 My point is, life is about balance. The good and the bad. The highs and the lows. The piña and the colada."

—ELLEN DEGENERES

# CHAPTER SEVEN

# Mood Changes and Difficult Behaviors

## BARB'S STORY

Jon has been married to Barb for 45 years. He has always adored her, and he is very devoted to caring for her, now that she is in the moderate stage of Alzheimer's disease. Over a year ago, their four children all contributed to a gift certificate to hire a housekeeper (Miss Ellen) to come four hours a week to help with the laundry and cleaning. When the gift certificate ran out, Jon made the decision to keep Miss Ellen coming to the house, mainly because she got along well with Barb, and Jon acknowledged that it had become "the girls' time" when she was there. He did have to reduce the time to three hours a week because it was expensive. Jon's children convinced him that it was money well spent, because Miss Ellen was helpful to both of them. She did laundry and cleaned the kitchen and bathroom for Jon. When Miss Ellen worked, she sang and visited with Barb, and after a few months, Jon felt comfortable leaving the house to get a little break. He usually did the grocery shopping, and if he had time, he would get a haircut. Over the past several months, however, Barb had started to say nasty things to Miss Ellen and question why she was at the house. Then, one day after Miss Ellen left, Barb accused Jon of having an affair with Miss Ellen. Jon was devasted by the accusation and didn't understand why his wife would say such terrible things. Jon would never, ever do anything to hurt his wife—he adored her.

# What to Expect

In the moderate stage of Alzheimer's disease, you may begin to notice greater changes in your loved one's personality and temperament. They may exhibit behaviors that are bizarre and even disturbing. Their mood may fluctuate without warning or provocation. The culprits behind these behaviors are the changes in the brain caused by the progression of the disease. These behaviors can be difficult to manage and understand, and, for caregivers, this can be devastating to watch.

"Challenging behaviors" is a general term used to describe a variety of actions related to the disease that may occur. Some of these behaviors can include anger, aggression, restlessness, and severe anxiety, as well as suspicion, paranoia, delusions, and hallucinations. Furthermore, there can be hypersexuality and disinhibition with an increase in poor judgment. This is not an exhaustive list; rather, these are some of the more common symptoms. It can be helpful to think about the sources that could be causing the behaviors to emerge, as they may be a result of physical or environmental triggers.

The most important part of understanding these behaviors is acknowledging that they are a method of communication. Challenging behaviors can indicate that your loved one is trying to tell you something. They are not trying to be difficult or acting this way on purpose. Alzheimer's disease has damaged the brain and, with that, inhibited your loved one's ability to communicate all that they are feeling and experiencing. Such challenging behaviors can occur when your loved one is trying to tell you, for example, that they are uncomfortable, embarrassed, self-conscious, or frightened. This disease has interrupted their ability to cope and respond to changing environments. Be patient and calm, and reassure your loved one in a loving, dignified way that you are there, they are safe, and everything is all right, even though you know that your loved one is having a great deal of difficulty in the moment. Try not to interpret difficult behaviors as a way of being noncompliant or troublesome or getting back at you. This is a devastating disease, so blame the disease, not your loved one. Aim to be strong and calm when your loved one is exhibiting challenging behaviors—this is exactly when they need your calm strength.

## ANGER AND AGGRESSION

Anger and aggression can manifest either verbally or physically, without warning or as a result of a complicated situation. Your loved one could be trying to communicate that they are overwhelmed, tired, uncomfortable, in pain, hot, cold, hungry, thirsty, or frustrated, to name a few possibilities.

Anxiety and restlessness can cause your loved one to pace or perseverate about something, such as wanting to go home or looking for their caregiver. Perhaps they are anxious around certain people, in crowds, or during transitions throughout the day. New environments, a recent hospitalization, or even recently moved furniture within the home can cause your loved one to become disorientated and unable to recognize their surroundings. Your loved one may feel alone, afraid, and fearful about their world. They may feel threatened and unsafe because of the uncertainty and confusion in their mind.

Your loved one might also become accusatory, suspicious, and delusional in this stage, making false claims about relationships or other fictional situations. For example, when Barb (see Barb's Story, page 89) accused Jon of having an affair with Miss Ellen, she truly believed that Jon was being unfaithful. Delusions in this context are beliefs that are firmly held about things or situations that are not real, as a result of Alzheimer's disease. If your loved one can't find something, such as papers, their purse, a watch, a hat, whatever—their untrue beliefs can lead them to accuse you or someone else of stealing or hiding it from them. Although these beliefs are of course not reality, they are very real for the person with the disease. They are trying so hard to make sense of their confusing world, yet their perceptions are off balance. Therefore, what they believe is not aligned with reality.

## HALLUCINATIONS

A similar but different symptom of Alzheimer's disease that your loved one may experience is hallucinations. Delusions are beliefs, whereas hallucinations stem from the sensory interpretations of situations or from the environment that your loved one is trying to understand. You may realize that your loved one sees, hears, smells, tastes, or feels something that isn't there. Hallucinations are false perceptions about people, objects, or events that involve the senses. For example, your loved one may see the face of a relative on the wall or a lampshade. They may have a conversation with someone who is not there. They may feel that they are holding hands with their partner or that the cat is sitting on their lap, when in reality, none of that is happening. Some hallucinations offer comfort to help your loved one cope with the confusing world they are experiencing. Other hallucinations can be scary or alarming for your loved one, and this may cause them to act out, perhaps putting themselves in danger, such as grabbing for a knife or trying to run away to "safety."

When hallucinations frighten your loved one, intervene calmly and immediately. Offer gentle reassurance, and explain that they are safe; you'll keep them safe and take care of them. Try to distract them by walking them into another room, turning on lights, or going for a walk. If they have a pet, have them stroke their furry friend to provide the physical sensations of comfort and support. Acknowledge their feelings and tell them that you know they are frightened, but they are safe. Offer them an item that brings them comfort, such as a favorite blanket or a newspaper, and gently touch their hand for reassurance.

Hallucinations, suspicion, and delusions are distressing for everyone involved. Be calm, try to figure out the triggers, and be ready to distract and calm your loved one when these episodes emerge.

## HYPERSEXUALITY AND OTHER EXTREMES

Some older adults may become disinhibited or experience hypersexuality. Disinhibition is a broad term for acting or speaking inappropriately without discretion or modesty. The individual may be socially or politically incorrect when interacting with others. They may say something that is racist, sexist, or otherwise offensive. Although it's simply a result of the disease, it can be horrifying to witness. Perhaps your loved one has started to flirt with others or even tried to grab or kiss someone. When this happens, the caregiver must intervene immediately. This can be done by telling their loved one, "That is not appropriate." Stating this out loud also helps diffuse the situation for others, as they see that you have taken charge of the situation. A gentle distraction and redirection for your loved one can help, and when possible, you can just leave the situation, offering a quiet apology and explanation to the person, who may not understand that your loved one has Alzheimer's disease. Those who understand that this can be part of the disease progression will hopefully not be offended or judgmental but, rather, sympathetic toward you, your loved one, and the situation.

## INSIDE ALZHEIMER'S

For the older adult in the moderate stage, their brain is experiencing the death of brain cells and the deterioration of the connections between them. Consequently, the functional ability of the older adult is getting significantly worse. The brain has areas of atrophy (the cells are dying), which are getting larger, and this is impacting more areas of the brain. At this stage, trying to walk in their shoes can be somewhat like driving or walking past a bad accident— you instinctively slow down to stop and look at it. Have you ever become so fixated on something that you couldn't look away or stop thinking about it? You can become all-consumed thinking about that experience or event. Now, picture yourself looking at that really bad accident, and know that you physically cannot walk away. You can't turn away from the gruesome scene for hours; in fact, you are compelled to stare at it without interruption. You become obsessed with the accident, and it grips every part of your existence. As this is happening, you begin to feel anxious and exhausted from the intensity of your fixation on the terrible situation. As your brain becomes fatigued, you start thinking strange thoughts that don't make sense, but you can't stop them from flooding your consciousness. Every part of yourself becomes enmeshed in the accident scene, trapping your thoughts and feelings and rendering you unable to articulate all that you're experiencing.

Eventually, something interrupts your fixation, and you are able to leave the disturbing scene. Exhausting, right? That is a brief glimpse into the world that your loved one is trying to manage, with a brain that is shrinking and unable to process all that is happening throughout their day.

## What to Say

As you struggle to interrupt your loved one's thought patterns, trying to communicate and reassure your loved one can be challenging. It's no easy task to change someone's mind when they have Alzheimer's.

However, some strategies can help you interrupt these negative thought patterns:

- Try to move your loved one into a different room.
- Speak in a calm, reassuring voice, even if your message sounds bizarre coming out of your mouth. Don't try to convince or argue with them, don't yell or belittle them. "Dad, put your pants back on—we need to go home now." Or, "Mom, Mr. Jones doesn't like to be kissed. Let's go into the kitchen and get some coffee."
- In the story of Jon and Barb, Jon learned to reply by reassuring Barb that he loves her and she is the only woman for him. Messages include, "I love you," "You're beautiful to me," and "Barb, you are the love of my life, it's okay. Everything's gonna be all right now." Jon has also learned to step outside and get some fresh air to keep himself calm and patient. He is so sad and overwhelmed by the accusations, but he has learned to try not to take it personally, as this is a disease that hurts the brain of the person he loves the most.

## What to Do

This can be a difficult part of the journey for the caregiver, as well as the person with Alzheimer's. Try to keep your perspective that this is a neurodegenerative disease that damages the brain over the course of many years. Try not to take it personally when your loved one is acting out. They are not trying to hurt you—when they blame you, it's because you are the one who is nearby. You are also the one taking care of your loved one, and sometimes being the caregiver requires you to make unpopular decisions. If you insist that your loved one is dressed properly or take them out of a situation when they behave inappropriately, they may lash out at you. Please know that when your loved one says hurtful things, that is simply the disease "talking" and negatively impacting their mood and behaviors.

Difficult behaviors are a method of communication. Strategies like distraction and redirection can be valuable when your loved one exhibits challenging behaviors. Try the following:

- Change the physical environment. Taking your loved one into another room or outside can cause a shift in perception, interrupting the cycle of the difficult thoughts or behavior.
- Distract them. Take a walk together, look at some pictures, turn on some music, or suggest another activity to interrupt their fragmented thought processes.
- Don't overreact; in fact, try to underreact. Be secure in knowing that the person accusing you of cheating or stealing is not the same person who you knew just a few years ago. Strive to be nonjudgmental—they need your love and support now more than ever.

### WHAT TO ASK THE DOCTOR

Keep bringing your notebook with your list of prepared questions for the doctor. Be honest in telling the doctor all that is happening with your loved one. If any topics are embarrassing for you or your loved one, make a list and hand it to the nurse. You can also request to meet privately to discreetly share your concerns.

Suggested questions might include:

- What medications or treatment options can help reduce difficult behaviors?
- How long could these behaviors last?
- If medication is prescribed, what side effects can we expect?
- How long before the medication will start working?
- When should we call or seek medical attention?

Be candid when talking to the doctor about your loved one. It is possible to simultaneously talk about the issues your loved one is having and still respect your loved one's dignity.

## Self-Care

Caregiving can be much like a roller-coaster ride, with ups and downs, twists and turns, and unexpected plunges into dark tunnels. Watching your loved one exhibit difficult behaviors can be devastating and overwhelming. If you've born the brunt of unfounded accusations and insults, this can surely test your tolerance and patience. By now, your loved one is in the moderate stage of Alzheimer's—it's the most challenging part of the disease.

Self-care is absolutely paramount when you are witnessing the decline of your loved one's personality. If you don't make time for yourself and prioritize self-care now, you may burn out, and then you won't do your best caregiving, and then you'll feel guilty. Breaks and downtime must become routine parts of the caregiving process. When you know that you'll have free time, this fact alone will help rejuvenate your spirit and allow you to better handle the more taxing parts of the caregiving journey.

Please don't go it alone—the burden can be overwhelming. When you take a break and allow someone else to be with your loved one, don't feel guilty. This is *your* medicine! Caregiver guilt can be paralyzing, and can prevent you from taking a much-needed break. You may think nobody else can do it like you, or that nobody knows your loved one like you do. That may be true, but there's no need to feel guilty—everyone deserves a break. Your love and devotion is the most precious gift of all, as you respect the dignity and quality of life of your loved one. Likewise, respecting your own quality of life requires that you take care of yourself, be gentle with yourself, and accept that you are special, too. If you need to cry, go ahead; if you need a belly laugh, find something to laugh about—you are human! Expressing yourself will help you make it through the challenging moments.

## JUST ONE THING

As you evolve through the long, complicated chapters of caregiving, you may become tired, frustrated, and worn down. If you can't go somewhere to recharge your batteries, just go outside. Get some mood-boosting vitamin D by sitting outside in the sun—even the wintertime sun offers benefits. Find a yoga or breathing exercise online, then do it. Shower and put on makeup. Look up quotes by the Dalai Lama or Oprah Winfrey or Maya Angelou or Eleanor Roosevelt, and savor their inspiring words. Seize the day, or, if all you have is a minute, seize that.

 Each person deserves a day away in which no problems are confronted, no solutions searched for. Each of us needs to withdraw from the cares which will not withdraw from us."

—MAYA ANGELOU

# CHAPTER EIGHT

# Step into Their World

## ROGER'S STORY, PART 1

Mia became the caregiver for her dad, Roger, when he was diagnosed with Alzheimer's disease. Even before the diagnosis, their relationship had always been somewhat strained. Part of the reason is that they were so much alike. Mia and her dad were both successful engineers, and Mia had inherited her dad's work ethic, attention to detail, and uncompromising personality. Mia's mom, Genny, is retired, but Mia became involved in the care of her dad when he became more difficult for her mom to manage alone. By that point, Roger had become very mean and refused EVERYTHING. Anytime assistance or a suggestion was offered, he said "NO!" Mia attended several caregiver support groups and learned that this was a normal part of the disease progression. If a person was always somewhat difficult, most likely this will continue into the disease process. There are other people who become very nice and pleasant as the disease progresses, but this wasn't the case for Roger. Mia quickly learned that his reactions were very consistent with his lifelong personality, and she would need to enlist creative approaches to get help for her parents.

## What to Expect

By now, you may have been involved with your loved one's care for several years. You may have adopting many routines and strategies to keep your loved one safe and at home. However, as new problems and deficits emerge, you may find that what's worked in the past does not work anymore. It can be trying as you attempt to figure out what the next steps should be.

There will come a time when using the bathroom becomes difficult for your loved one to manage. Some people simply forget to use the bathroom and become incontinent. Others may still feel the urge to go, but don't know how to get to the bathroom or pull down their pants and undergarments, and then, after emptying their bladder or bowels, they may forget to clean themselves. Think about all the steps that we take for granted every time we need to use the bathroom. This process can become complicated and overwhelming for those with diminished cognitive ability, memory loss, and confusion. The same set of functional challenges can also interfere with your loved one's ability to get dressed. For example, they may put their underpants on over their pants. They may no longer remember to put a bra on, or know how to fasten it. Shirts may be buttoned incorrectly. Your loved one may choose clothing that is not appropriate for the season; perhaps they'll choose a long-sleeved shirt, sweatshirt, and coat when the weather is in the 80s. Or they'll put on a summer dress when the temperature is below zero. These are the moments in which caregivers need to be inventive, for safety's sake.

Mia learned that her dad was more amenable to getting dressed when he thought he was going to work. On the days he refused to get dressed, Mia and Genny told him that he must get ready for work or he would be late. Genny would lay out his clothes and help him "look nice for work." They told Roger it was business casual at work and he didn't need to wear his suit. This strategy worked for many months, although Genny had to learn to let go of the guilt that she felt every time she told Roger that he was going to work.

This type of creative storytelling is also called therapeutic fibbing or telling therapeutic "fiblets." These are the stories you tell your loved one to help them complete the tasks essential to their well-being. Telling Roger that he was going to work was not done with the intention of deceit—rather, it motivated him to put on clean clothes and allowed Genny to help him with bathing and grooming. As a result, he would shower and allow Genny to shave him about twice each week. Prior to their discovery of therapeutic fibbing, Roger would refuse to shower or shave or weeks. He gave Genny a hard time and was nasty to her. When Genny modified her approach and shifted the focus onto helping him "get ready for work," he didn't give her a hard time. After Roger was "ready for work," they would eat breakfast together, and Roger would read the paper and forget all about going to work. If he did insist on going to work, Genny would take him out for a drive, and they would run some errands or visit the local mall for a walk. This was a very successful intervention; however, it was exhausting for Genny. Over time, Mia became more involved to help out her mom.

## INCREASED DEPENDENCY

As your loved one is unable to do as much for themselves, it's important to help them do as much as they still can, with as much independence as possible. For example, say your loved one forgets to go to the bathroom, but when they do remember, they can still go independently. Offer prompting with gentle reminders to use the bathroom throughout the day. Set a timer to go off every two hours as a reminder to go to the bathroom; this can help minimize "accidents." This is a commonly used strategy in adult day programs, assisted living facilities, and skilled nursing homes.

Offering reminders that help assist with the activities of daily living, such as taking medication, drinking water, and going to the bathroom, can simplify caregiving. More importantly, they will help keep your loved one free from unnecessary and harmful complications like becoming dehydrated or making medication errors.

As the level of dependency increases, your responsibilities of caregiving will increase as well. In the effort to maintain balance with respect to your loved one's dignity and quality of life, consider how you can help them feel comfortable and capable in different areas of their life. Yes, Alzheimer's disease has changed your loved one's brain, but you are in the position to help them feel empowered with meaning and purpose. Being dependent and relying on others can be devastating for your loved one, even as they experience increased cognitive impairment. You have the unique opportunity to help them feel special and valued by treating them as such.

## CHANGES IN EATING

Your loved one may have difficulty using the proper utensils when eating. Allow them to use a spoon instead of a fork, if that's easier; this retains their dignity by allowing them to eat independently. Finger foods are nice, as they can be eaten independently. Some people may have little or no difficulty using utensils well into the moderate stage of the disease. Whatever the menu, if you include a variety of healthy foods, you'll help your loved one meet their nutritional needs. If they experience a decrease or other changes in appetite, offer small quantities of healthy food frequently throughout the day.

## WANDERING

Approximately 60 percent of all people with Alzheimer's disease will wander at some point during the course of the disease. This is a very serious occurrence that requires immediate attention. There are safety devices that your loved one can wear, such as GPS watches, emergency medical alert bracelets, Life Alert, and other products that are available regionally. There are also some specialized programs available in certain regions of the country that provide tracking assistance if your loved one wanders, like Project Lifesaver. Check with your local county office for aging or local chapter of the Alzheimer's Association for a list of available products. Roger (see Roger's Story, Part 1, page 99) started wandering recently; in fact, one day, he walked out of the house and was gone for three hours. A friend of Mia's found Roger at the local gas station. He had soiled himself and was disoriented and upset. Genny got Roger home, and he kept saying, "We need to go to the bank." Genny reassured him that the banking had been done and he needed to stay home now. The more that Genny tried to orient him, the more upset Roger became. Roger kept saying that he had to go out, and Mia, who had just arrived, said, "Dad, I went to the bank for you—here's the receipt." She pulled out a receipt from her lunch. It calmed Roger down to have that receipt in his hands.

Stepping into their world will help you manage and understand some of the wildly unpredictable events that can occur as a result of the disease. Creative and vigilant thinking is key to both peace and safety.

Think about installing locks that are out of your loved one's view on every door that leads outside. Talk to the doctor about medication that may help reduce anxiety and your loved one's need to wander.

### INSIDE ALZHEIMER'S DISEASE

Your loved one may have an increase in poor judgment and may no longer be oriented to time and place. As you know, Alzheimer's disease destroys the cells in the brain that communicate with each other. When parts of the brain can't send and receive messages, the systems of communication break down. Roger wandered out of the house again when Genny was taking a shower. By stepping into Roger's shoes and thinking about what he would do, Genny found him calmly walking down the road. When she questioned him, he explained that he was going to see his grandpa. Roger had grown up in a village on the outskirts of a small city, and most of his relatives lived within a couple of blocks of each other. In his childhood, it was common for Roger to walk to see his relatives. Now, all these years later, Roger was thinking about his childhood and even believed he was in that time and place. Back then, walking to see his grandpa was perfectly normal. But now, this long-term memory has triggered wandering, which is of course very dangerous for Roger, who could get lost or walk out into traffic.

As you step into your loved one's shoes, think about why something is happening. Why are they resisting? Why are they insisting? Consider the possibilities, ask them their thoughts, and then join in their reality to accomplish whatever needs to be done to achieve a peaceful and safe resolution, even if it includes some "fiblets."

## What to Say

Let's explore the dos and don'ts of what to say when these types of situations arise. Let's say your dad insists on seeing his grandpa:

- DO say that he'll be coming over at dinnertime or that you'll be seeing him Sunday.

- DON'T try to orient your loved one to reality. Saying, "Dad, Grandpa died 15 years ago" could momentarily devastate your loved one, potentially triggering feelings of grief, loss, and fear.
- DON'T try to "snap them out of it." Families often think, "If I could just get him to understand what's going on right now, if I explain what's happening, he'll get it." That will not happen with Alzheimer's disease. The more you try to explain what is happening and try to orient them, the more complicated the situation will become.
- DO remain calm, gentle, and kind, with sensitivity to your loved one's feelings. This will minimize negative emotions, reduce fear, and contribute to feelings of comfort and safety.

## What to Do

After Roger wandered away and Mia's friend found him, Mia decided to find a program to help keep her dad safe. At a caregiver support group, she learned about a registry monitored by the county sheriff's office that has the names and pictures of people of all ages who are at risk for wandering. Mia registered Roger and put her own name down as the primary contact. Mia also helped Genny make some changes in their home to reduce the chances of Roger wandering again. They hung long panels that look like bookcases on the back of all of the doors to the outside. When Roger looks at the door, it looks like a bookcase to him now. Mia also installed a slide lock at the top of the door, just out of Roger's sight, so he can't open the door. Genny uses the lock when she's in the shower or not able to keep her eyes on Roger. Additional ideas might include:

- Installing grab bars in the bathroom to assist your loved one with stability and reduce the risk of falling. This can also reduce your own risk of being injured if you assist with lifting and moving your loved one.
- Learning about local programs and services that can benefit your loved one and provide you the opportunity to take a break.

- Spending time learning about resources, sifting through what is useful at the moment, and noting what you may need in the future. Then, you'll be ready when you need to put services in place to enhance your and your loved one's quality of life.
- Coordinating services. If you are unable to provide the hands-on care to help with bathing or toileting, seek out these types of services in your area.
- Networking. Ask for the help of others to look for information on your loved one's behalf about programs and services that may be beneficial.

It can be a lifesaver to learn as much as you can about the disease, how it impacts your loved one, and what you can do to help. As you experiment with interventions and strategies, you'll develop a keen awareness about how your loved one reacts in certain situations. And when you step into their world, you'll more easily come up with creative solutions to meet their needs and keep them safe.

## WHAT TO ASK THE DOCTOR

Of course, you'll bring your trusty notebook with your questions written down in advance! List any changes in behavior or health that need to be discussed with the doctor. Include an up-to-date list of all medications, supplements, and dosages. As always, be honest and open about the changes you and your loved one are facing. Speak privately if needed. Some issues to cover might include:

- If you're having trouble getting your loved one to bathe and shave, or other self-care activities, do they have any suggestions?
- How often do they really need a full shower? Will sponge baths suffice?
- How do I get my loved one to wear disposable undergarments?
- Are there any medications that can help at this stage?
- Are there other interventions or strategies that will help?

# Self-Care

As the months and even years add up when you're caregiving, taking care of yourself must continue to be a priority. Carve time out of your busy life—this time invested in you is well spent. It's imperative, just as you care for your loved one, to care for yourself. Sometimes this means letting go of your tight grip on the reins that you've become so accustomed to. If your loved one is having a bad day, let it go. If they insist on eating toast for breakfast and lunch, let it go. As long as it doesn't happen every day, try to let things go. Ask for help to let someone else come in so you can get a much-needed break. Easier said than done, indeed! The more your loved one depends on you emotionally and physically, and the more care you provide, the greater your risk for getting sick or injured. Even if you're tired, try to exercise; moving just a little more can help reduce stress. You may also need to rest or take a nap—probably many naps, just to catch up. Retreating from the stress and burden of caregiving is essential to your well-being, as is relaxation. If you become run down or get injured, who will step in? Taking care of yourself can actually prevent a crisis. When you think about it that way, you'll realize that self-care is one of the best investments you can make in yourself and your loved one.

## JUST ONE THING

Mark your calendar for you! Yes, breaks from the demands of caregiving should ideally be scheduled on a regular basis. Take a moment each day to appreciate all that you do and have done for your loved one. You are an incredible gift; you have given so generously of yourself, your energy, and your patience. Take a break to nourish your spirit, rejuvenate your soul, and appreciate how far you've come on this journey. Snuggle up in your favorite blanket or stretch out on a lawn chair. Take some deep breaths and enjoy a moment of gratitude. Try to think about something or someone you're grateful for. It doesn't need to be complicated or take a long time. Gratitude can help your heart smile again by revisiting all that matters to you. Being grateful is not a cliché or a trendy idea; rather, it's a rare opportunity to stop and catch your breath and simply be, if only for a moment.

 Gratitude makes sense of our past, brings peace for today, and creates a vision for tomorrow." **–MELODY BEATTIE**

# CHAPTER NINE

# Changing Care Needs

## ROGER'S STORY, PART 2

As the situation has worsened, Roger requires more care, and Mia is very concerned about Genny as well. The previous month, Genny slipped and fell in the bathroom and broke her shoulder. At the time, Genny was helping Roger, who was having terrible diarrhea. The diarrhea was a side effect from the medication that was prescribed by an urgent care center. They didn't have his medical history, and Genny was exhausted from taking care of him, so she forgot to mention that certain antibiotics caused Roger to have diarrhea.

When Genny fell, she was able to crawl to the phone and call 911. The ambulance came and took both of them to the hospital when Genny told them that Roger could not be left home alone. Genny was admitted—her fracture would require surgery to repair; she also had a mild concussion. Roger was placed in the emergency department with no understanding about the condition of his wife. He wanted to leave and repeatedly asked to go home. Over and over he asked to go home. Some of the medical staff understood that Roger had Alzheimer's disease; others did not.

Mia was out of the country for work when she got the call that both of her parents were in the hospital. She booked an emergency flight home. While waiting at the airport for her flight, she made arrangements for her dad to go to an assisted living facility for emergency respite. Coincidentally, about six months prior, Genny got the flu and Mia decided to tour a "continuing care community" with the thought that this might be an option for her dad if something were to happen to her mom. Mia called the director of admissions from the airport, who contacted the intake coordinator at the hospital's emergency department. After 72 hours, Roger was qualified for admission into the assisted living facility. With Roger safe in assisted living, Mia could focus on her mom and the imminent surgery.

# What to Expect

It can be very difficult to know what the right decision should be, since Alzheimer's disease looks different for every person. Furthermore, it's experienced differently by every family. As your loved one moves through the moderate stage of the disease, their functional decline could be very severe. For some, serious physical limitations may accompany the memory loss and cognitive impairment. Others may still be in fairly good physical health but have profound cognitive impairment. In either case, the caregiver generally takes on a higher level of responsibility.

Making decisions is one of the most controversial parts of being the primary caregiver. When decisions are made, not everyone will be happy with the outcome. Mia made the decision to place her dad in a safe setting while her mom recuperated. She has a brother who is estranged from the family and lives across the country, and so she was able to make this decision on her own (though there were some moments of friction following Genny's return home, as described on the next page). However, for many families, especially when multiple family members are involved in the decision-making process, it can lead to a full-blown war if everyone does not agree on the care plan. Getting everyone to agree can be complicated and stressful. All you can do in cases like this is to keep your focus on what best meets the needs of your loved one.

## CHANGING CARE NEEDS

When a higher level of care is required, decisions need to be made based on who is available to assist with care and whether the loved one's needs can be met in the current setting. If 24/7 care or supervision is needed, can the family provide that? Or, can someone coordinate the hiring of workers to come in to help, and then the family can fill in the care gaps?

Could someone move in to help assist with the care of the loved one? Approximately 70 percent of all people who have Alzheimer's disease are cared for in the home. Many families want their loved one to be at home, but this may not work in all cases. Many caregivers still work, or they are not able to provide the level of care needed.

## WHEN THE CAREGIVER GETS SICK OR INJURED

It's important to be realistic about the type of care that your loved one requires. Try to have a backup plan if something should happen to you. Then, test out that plan. Bring in someone else to be with your loved one so you can take a break from the situation. Don't wait for the crisis to happen. Now is the time to identify who will assist when you're not available.

When Mia visited her dad at the assisted living facility, he was very upset. He was cranky and complained about everything. He didn't understand what happened to Genny, and didn't even ask about her until Mia brought it up. Although they didn't always get along, her parents were devoted to each other. But now, Roger acted as though he didn't even know who Genny was. That was very troubling to Mia. Interestingly, according to the staff, after Mia had left, Roger was pleasant and was no trouble for the staff to manage at all. He ate his meals, took his medication, and even attended activities.

A few days after Genny's surgery, she was released from the hospital and set up with support services to help her recuperate, including physical and occupational therapy. However, when she got home, she was upset that Roger was not there. She didn't understand why Mia couldn't arrange care for him at home, as the assisted facility was not covered by insurance and was quite expensive.

Mia knew that her mom was upset because she could no longer take care of Roger. After 50 years of being together, she was devastated at the thought of being separated from him. Mia decided to move in with her mom temporarily so she could help her recover from the surgery and drive her to see Roger as often as possible. Initially, Roger didn't recognize Genny, but then she began to sing their favorite song. She held his hand and he smiled lovingly at her. It was a special moment for

Genny. Life had changed so much for them, Genny thought. She didn't know how to get Roger home. If he stays in the facility, she thought, their life savings will be gone in less than a year.

After four months, Genny and Mia brought Roger back home, and Mia coordinated care for both of her parents. A home health aide came in for three hours each day to help with care, meals, and housework. The family was eligible for a program provided by their county's office for aging that subsidized 60 percent of the cost of the aide visits. This plan worked for about eight months, but then Roger got sick and needed full-time care. At this point, he needed to be fed and no longer recognized Genny or Mia. There were so many transitions over the past several years that had to be managed. Genny had gotten worn down, due to the increased level of care her husband required. Genny and Mia started to tour a few nursing homes in the event that they could no longer provide care for him.

It's important to have a backup plan. Come up with a list of people who can be called upon in your absence, or have a facility in mind that could temporarily provide care for your loved one.

## ACCEPTING HELP

It can be a lifeline to bring more care into the home. Extra hands on board, especially expert ones, will enable your loved one to remain at home longer and reduce your burden. This is a very hard time for your family, and it can be devastating to realize that you may not be able to provide the necessary care to keep your loved one at home.

When you accept help, this shows that you actually have immense strength by demonstrating that you'll allow someone to step in. Ask a cooperative sibling, a member of the faith community, or a niece or nephew or grandchild if they can help, even if it's just to take your loved one out for lunch or for a drive once in a while.

The challenge is to be prepared to see that things may be done differently than you would do them. Initially, this may make you feel anxious. If your helper opens the bedroom window and lets some cool air in the house and you feel it's drafty, let it go—maybe the house smells a little and you don't even recognize it. If your helper takes your loved one out for coffee and together they stop and take a short walk in the park, try not to worry. Tell your helper what your loved one is able to do and what is more challenging for them, and explain any safety risks up front.

Maybe you've been responsible for so long, you've forgotten how to let go a little. Yes, you definitely know what's best, and you are by far the expert about your loved one. However, letting go and allowing someone else to help in a different way may bring great pleasure to your loved one. If it's not perfect—maybe they had ice cream for lunch—let it go and enjoy your free time. The next time your helper wants to give them ice cream for lunch, suggest that they have something more substantial first, if that would be okay. Resist the urge to criticize—don't lose your helper! You need and deserve the break.

## CAREGIVER GUILT

When you accept help, the secret to freely accepting the help is to not feel guilty. Dare to acknowledge that you actually need to get out for a while. You are not a robot! You are a human, and you can become very isolated as you dedicate so much of your time and energy to someone else. You are coordinating their care, making meals, managing meds, going to doctor appointments, doing laundry, or overseeing all of this. All the while, you're watching your loved one deteriorate before your very eyes. This can be a lonely time in your life. Breaks and rest will make the situation more bearable for you and your loved one.

Maybe you just don't know where to start. If someone offers to help and you don't know how to factor them in, make a list. When you identify a need, write it in your notebook with the date, then add it to the list for others to see. Be specific; that way, people will know exactly how they can help. Ideas might include:

*"I could use help with cutting the grass (or shoveling snow)."*

*"Dad's favorite meal is spaghetti. Would you be willing to make it? What, you'll do it every other Sunday?! Thank you!"*

*"Mom and Dad would like to go to their worship service. They need a ride on Saturdays."*

*"Dad could really use a ride to the senior center on Mondays and Wednesdays when I'm at work; that way, he won't be home alone all day."*

Think it's hard? Think you can't say yes? When caregiver guilt sneaks in or does a full-on stampede on your heart and emotions, take a moment and think about all of the good that you've done. The sheer recognition of your time, love, devotion, and commitment can help to reduce feelings of caregiver guilt. Some people with Alzheimer's disease can become manipulative and pour on the guilt. Perhaps they've been that way their entire life. Once again, be brave, and remember that when you take care of yourself, you are better able to take care of your loved one. Surely, you don't want to become bitter and resentful about your caregiving role; taking breaks and accepting help will protect you against negative feelings and emotions that will take a toll on your spirit and trickle down to your loved one.

## FAMILY DIFFERENCES

Your loved one may need to downsize and move into a smaller living space. Moving is rarely easy, but simplifying can help your loved one age safely at home. These kinds of transitions can be very helpful in planning for the future. Start the conversation early; don't delay.

As the disease progresses, some families experience a tremendous amount of conflict around financial decisions. A family fighting over money and resources is nothing new. This is when being a caregiver can become especially intense and stressful. Make sure you know the wishes of your loved one.

Sometimes, families must spend money to bring help into the home. In Roger's Story, Part 2 (page 109), the family had to pay for assisted living while Genny recuperated, but this was money well spent. Indeed, some family members may flip out and start a fight when the subject of money comes up, even for providing care or equipment for your loved one. Other family members will be supportive. Work with the family members or friends who will support you. When you must interact with a person who is not supportive, keep it to a minimum. Maybe they don't need to be included in every decision, especially if you know they'll give you a hard time. Families can be the greatest source of support— or strain.

## INSIDE ALZHEIMER'S

Keeping your loved one safe and well cared for should always be the guiding force. As their brain continues to shrink, your loved one will become more impaired and need additional care and support. Being dependent on others can evoke feelings of anger or sadness in that person. Conversely, your loved one may not understand all that they have lost. It's up to you, as the caregiver, to help your loved one feel safe, secure, and loved. Walking in their shoes, imagine yourself getting very upset while you're walking on a path in the woods, then accidentally straying from the path and getting lost. You have no food or water, and it's getting dark. No one knows where you are, and you're surrounded by trees and darkness. You're becoming overwhelmed and upset, your heart is racing, you're sweating and cold at the same time, and now you're breathing faster. Then, out of the darkness, someone gently takes your hand and guides you out of the woods toward a room. You start feeling warmer when they give you a blanket. They put a cup of tea in your hands and put a something on a plate next to you. Your heart rate slows, and you begin to feel calmer and warmer. You know you are safe now.

## What to Say

As a caregiver, you may know what needs to happen—or maybe you haven't got a clue. Throughout this journey, continue asking questions about what type of care your loved one needs right now, as well as what they'll need in the future. Should they move out of their home? Should you or someone else move in with them? Care transitions can be some of the biggest decisions you'll make. Here's how you can approach them:

*"Mom, we all think it's time to have Barb move in with you to help out for a while."*

*"Mom, moving into a smaller apartment will be easier for you to manage, and you'll be closer to us."*

*"Dad, can we start to get rid of some of the clutter around here? We're worried about you tripping and falling."*

*"Dad, if we don't clean out this clutter, you may trip and fall, and we don't want you to end up in the hospital."*

*"Mom and Dad, when you accept a little help, you'll be able to manage the home longer. You want 100 percent of your freedom and independence, but if you allow us to help with 10 percent of your responsibilities, then you'll still have 90 percent of your independence. We want you to live at home together, but Dad, as Mom needs more care, we need to make sure that you can manage it all."*

When families argue over possessions, you can say, "Mom, we can put a label on everything, and then you can decide who gets what."

The defining factor, which will help you always remember the top priority when faced with tough discussions, is that your loved one must be safe and have care or supervision. When you have these conversations, enlist the support of those people who will help.

## What to Do

When you're helping your loved one with a physical task, such as buttoning their shirt, it's important to talk to them. When your loved one felt lost in the woods and a gentle hand guided them out to safety, that was you! Yours is the hand that guides them out of the scary place and makes them feel comforted. Your kindness, patience, and calm and loving approach can be lifelines, especially when a situation is spiraling out of control or your loved one is upset and disoriented. That said, having someone help us in the bathroom is contrary to human nature. It's uncomfortable and awkward, so, even now, do whatever you can to maintain your loved one's dignity and treat them with the respect they deserve.

While you're still actively caring for your loved one, it's smart to start touring a few long-term care facilities and look at their ratings online. If you have a few places in mind, it will be easier to execute a plan if a crisis occurs. Do everything you can to prevent hasty decisions. Gather information and keep it just in case you need it. It may not be necessary or even beneficial to include the entire family. However, you can have some ideas ready for when you do decide to talk to others involved. For example, "I've toured some facilities and three of them have a great rating. Would you like to hear more?"

For most families, keeping their loved one at home is the only decision, and there is no other option. If this is the case, you'll need to find an agency that helps provide care, or privately hire a friend of the family or other trusted person to help out. If you do bring in people to help care for your loved one, lock up all medications, cash, checks, and valuables. Many agencies do a fantastic job of screening their employees; others do not. Take some basic precautions to protect your loved one and their identity and assets.

In talking to your loved one, keep your messages short and sweet. Reassure them that you're doing everything you can to make them comfortable, happy, and safe. For Mia, Genny, and Roger, when Roger did come home, Genny held his hand as they sat on the porch, and she sang him their favorite song. Roger smiled lovingly at Genny. He couldn't say her name anymore, but he knew that he was loved.

Like the saying, "No good deed goes unpunished," there will be many moments when you'll be unpopular with your loved one and other family members. If you keep safety and care the highest priorities, you'll know in your heart that you've done well and will continue to do your very best, and everyone else will just have to adjust.

## WHAT TO ASK THE DOCTOR

Because you can't imagine going to an appointment without it, you will surely have your notebook, complete with your latest questions, changes in behavior and ability, and current medications and dosages all written down in advance. Questions you might want to address include:

- What happens when they become incontinent?
- Is my loved one declining?
- Are the current medications still needed and beneficial? Are there new ones you might consider, in light of recent changes?
- Is it time to move to a higher level of care?
- How can we modify the environment to keep our loved one safe?
- How can I get them to drink enough water? How much do they need?
- Doctor, do you have any other suggestions or comments?

# Self-Care

As the chapters of caregiving start to add up, several years may have passed on this journey. It's truly like running a marathon, not a sprint. With it, you have moments of energy and times of exhaustion and complete despair. This is when self-care can rescue you. Taking a break and getting away from the situation will rejuvenate your spirit. You're only human, and it always takes more than one person to provide care for someone with Alzheimer's disease. Please get some help. Genny tried to manage everything on her own, it became overwhelming, and then she got injured.

Go for a walk, get a fancy coffee or latte with your best friend. Meet your buddy for a game of golf—nine holes, just a quick round. Self-care is the antidote to isolation and despair. You deserve a break; you've more than earned some time for yourself. Please don't martyr yourself; it's not necessary or healthy for anyone involved. As someone who has witnessed hundreds of Alzheimer's caregiver experiences, I can say with certainty: **Regular self-care will help you make it through this marathon of caregiving.**

## JUST ONE THING

When you're running a marathon, you need to get some water along the way, right? Likewise, you must do something for yourself to keep your spirits going, no matter how small. Why not make it a culinary something? Host a little ceremony for yourself, complete with a big mug of hot chocolate with whipped cream, or a tall glass of sweet tea with a slice of fresh lemon. Feed your spirit and nourish your soul in whatever way does the trick. Indulge yourself with your favorite chocolate dessert or an ice cream cone. Chances are good that you haven't taken a moment to enjoy something special that you absolutely *love*. Maybe your favorite dessert is a cannoli or baklava, or maybe you're craving a plate of spaghetti and meatballs at your favorite little bistro. If you can't eat out, order it to go, take it home, put it on a special plate, and enjoy.

Remember those little things that you love. They may have gotten lost among the chores, the decisions, and the appointments. Treat yourself; you deserve it, and it will literally and figuratively feed your spirit.

> " Indulgence comes in all varieties: a mouthful of gourmet chocolate, a hot stone massage, a week in Paris, or 20 uninterrupted minutes to get lost in a book."
>
> —GINA GREENLEE

# PART THREE
# LATE STAGE

As the disease progresses into the late-middle stages, and then ultimately into the final stage, we'll explore some of the things you and your loved one may experience. We'll also cover some practical tips and strategies that can help you navigate common situations that can occur on this part of the journey. The end stage of Alzheimer's disease can last for just a few months or up to two years. This has been a long journey, but knowledge has been your ally all along, and it will continue to serve you as you make thoughtful and informed choices on behalf of your loved one and yourself.

# CHAPTER TEN

# Embracing the Moment

## ROSIE'S STORY

Rosie was the matriarch of her large family. She gave birth to seven children and took in three foster children as well. Rosie was married to Vincent for 55 years before he passed away from pancreatic cancer 11 years ago. After Vincent died, the family quickly noticed that Rosie had become confused, disoriented, and was suddenly terrified to stay at home alone. The family thought Rosie was suffering from overwhelming grief over the loss of Vincent. After several months and multiple medical evaluations, Rosie was diagnosed with Alzheimer's disease. Looking back, the family realized that Vincent had been covering and caring for Rosie for many years, even as she became more confused and had memory loss. In the 11 years since her diagnosis, the family has managed to take care of Rosie and keep her at home, but now Rosie is in the final stage of Alzheimer's disease.

## What to Expect

Your loved one will need full care, and along with that, they'll continue to need your unconditional love and support. Their needs have changed, and their dependence on you will reach a new level. Your caregiving role is changing yet again, and you'll need to continue to be flexible, honest, and deeply committed to maintaining your loved one's dignity and quality of life.

In this chapter, we'll cover many common issues that can occur at the end stage of the disease, including:

- Anticipatory grief
- Letting go
- Finding joy in the moment
- Being fully present with your loved one

## ANTICIPATORY GRIEF

Throughout the progression of the disease, you've watched over your loved one, caring for them and keeping them safe. Over time, you've learned to adjust your approach and modify your expectations. And, unfortunately, in all of this, you've watched your loved one deteriorate and change from who they once were, and your world will never be the same.

Caregiving can trigger negative or complicated feelings caused by watching your loved one suffer, struggle, and transform over time, and knowing that you can't stop this devastating disease. It's very normal for caregivers to feel emotions related to grief and loss. You may have heard of the stages of grief: denial, anger, guilt, sadness, and acceptance. People don't necessarily experience these emotions in that exact order, and you can move in and out of stages as time passes—grief is experienced differently by everyone. Just know that, no matter how you are feeling, your caregiving has been a precious gift to your loved one. Think about all the good that you've done! When no one is looking, you care for your loved one. When you're feeling the loss, make sure to face your feelings, but also be sure to take time to consider all the good you've done. You've helped them when they needed it the most and provided them with care, comfort, and the best quality of life they could have asked for.

## LETTING GO

The reality of caring for a loved one with Alzheimer's is that you are forced to let go, a little at a time, through all the stages of the disease. Through the early and middle stages, you've adjusted to each new decline. Now, as you're facing the end stage of the disease, think about letting go of any guilt, exhaustion, or anger, and try to find some peace in your heart. Maybe you need to let go physically and allow someone else to help when it requires a team of people to provide care. Whether your "letting go" is emotional or physical, you can still do so much to keep your loved one comfortable and in good care.

## FINDING JOY IN THE MOMENT

Look for moments when you can find a reason to smile with your loved one. If you can't seem to find any, create one. Pull out some photos, talk about a special memory, and create moments of joy in being together. Living in the present moment allows you to relax and experience the sights, sounds, and feelings that emerge when you take a moment and focus on the positive. Have a cup of tea together, watch the birds through the window, or sit outside and breathe the fresh air. Finding joy can last a moment or longer, but the sense of peace and connectedness it provides is enduring.

### INSIDE ALZHEIMER'S

In the late stages of Alzheimer's disease, the brain continues to shrink, causing tissue damage and nerve cell death. By now, the damage to the brain is extensive, and most areas of the brain have been affected by the disease. Your loved one may lose the ability to communicate and to care for themselves. They may lose the ability to control facial expressions; this can make communication difficult at times. It can be tough to know what they are feeling, so stepping into their shoes might involve some guesswork. As an example, if you were sitting in a reclining chair 20 hours a day, napping most of that time, in the moments when you're awake, what would you like to look at? What would make you happy? Think about those same questions for your loved one—consider what would make them happy and content.

## BEING FULLY PRESENT WITH YOUR LOVED ONE

Finding joy in the moment leads you directly to being fully present with your loved one. As you sit together, resist thinking about chores, tasks, appointments, planning meals, coordinating care, paying bills, the future—all of it. This doesn't need to be complicated. When you simply direct your full attention to thinking about a fond memory, something that you appreciate, or just being together now, this will allow you the gift of being fully present in the moment.

# What to Say

As you interact with your loved one in the severe stage, continue to talk to them, speak to them with love and respect, and explain what you may be doing. You can simply vocalize your thoughts:

> *"Hi Mom—I'm opening the window up, just a little, to let some fresh air in for you. Here, have a sip of water and I'll bring you a snack."*

> *"Mom, let's go out on the porch. It's really nice out this afternoon."*
> *(You can make sure they're comfortable and then sit alongside them.)*

> *"Here, Dad, look at this picture of us when we went swimming. That was fun, going to the lake in the summer." (If he doesn't respond, just smile and tell him how much fun you all had together.)*

Keep the conversation pleasant and upbeat, and try to be authentic. There's no need to act differently or pretend to be someone that you're not. When you're having a bad day, be honest, but try to resist talking to your loved one about being sad or upset.

> *"Honey, I'm having a bad day today—let's just sit quietly and watch a movie."*

> *"I'm sorry I'm a little cranky today. Good thing we have each other."*

# What to Do

In the end stage of the disease, you may need to make some changes in the care plan. This may include making additional changes to the home environment. If your loved one is having difficulty with mobility and walking becomes a challenge, you may need to move their bed to a room that's closer to a bathroom. Less walking will help reduce the chances of falling. Adapt the environment based on their abilities or lack thereof. Preventing falls is a priority at this stage, as the disease has impacted all areas of their life.

When they become incontinent and confined to bed, ideally, you'll still want the bathroom near your loved one to help you manage disposal of urination and bowel movements. At this point, it's important to keep them clean and dry to protect their skin from infections. If you give sponge baths, be as thorough as possible in both washing and drying and inspect their body for irritations or infections. Try to keep them in a warm, draft-free location as they dry.

It's important for caregivers to know about pressure ulcers, otherwise known as bedsores. Bedsores are a common issue; they can be prevented, but, if early signs of damage are not noticed, they can get worse and become very painful or infected. A pressure ulcer or bedsore is an area of skin, and sometimes also the tissue underneath, that has become damaged because of pressure. These may develop over bony areas that are close to the skin. The bedsore can form because the blood supply to the skin is reduced, and the skin becomes starved of oxygen and nutrients. Sitting or lying in the same position for too long is a common cause of this painful condition.

Especially as it progresses, Alzheimer's disease increases the risk of pressure ulcers, because your loved one may have difficulty with mobility and walking; even poor diet and dehydration can weaken the skin and lessen its ability to heal itself. Incontinence can cause moisture from leaks, and this too, can damage the skin. Difficulty in communicating may make it hard for your loved one to tell you they are in pain or want to move. Your role as a thoughtful and perceptive caregiver is vital to keeping your loved one comfortable and safe as these kinds of issues become a possibility.

You can help prevent bedsores by making sure your loved one doesn't spend all their time lying in one position. Turn them if necessary. If they are cognizant of your efforts, sit on one side of their bed one day, then switch to the other side the next day so they are forced to turn their body. You can also move a small television from side to side each day.

At this point, spouses may also need to start sleeping in a different room. Maybe it's time to bring in a hospital bed. If your partner becomes incontinent, they may soil the sheets and linens. Getting a hospital bed for the home may help meet the changing needs of your loved one. A hospital bed will allow your loved one to sit up, and this will help with feeding and drinking fluids. It's a little easier to help your loved one out of a hospital bed, since you can simply swing their legs around as opposed to having to get them up from a flat-lying position in a regular bed. A hospital bed must be ordered by the physician and be medically necessary for insurance to cover it. However, adaptive equipment like this will help you provide a higher level of care and prevent you from getting injured when trying to move or assist your loved one.

Watching a loved one deteriorate can be very stressful for families. As the caregiver, part of your role may be to keep the peace among family members. Sometimes families will fight, due to the increased tension and stress during this time. You may need to brainstorm some conflict-reducing strategies in effort to maintain peace. Commit to being the voice of reason—someone needs to be!

When changes and decisions need to be made, these can be the times that families argue most.

Here are some common conflict-reducing strategies:

- Have a conversations in which you all agree to listen to other's opinions calmly.
- If conflict erupts, choose the high road; refuse engage in an argument.
- Watch your tone and volume. Remember how shouting and yelling near your loved one can be very upsetting for them.

- Try to be flexible whenever possible—how important is the argument?
- Always keep in mind what makes your loved one happy, content, and able to receive excellent care.

Keep the focus on your loved one, not family drama. This mind-set will help guide the difficult decisions that need to be made. This will also set the tone for peaceful resolution and help keep you connected to your loved one.

Also, focus on the positive whenever possible. Look at the positive work you've done—the commitment you've made and the journey you've traveled is time well spent. When you focus on the positive, it will help you carve out opportunities to find the joy in this part of the journey. Concentrating on the positive will allow you to be fully present with your loved one in those moments when they need your companionship, love, and reassurance the most. When you decide to focus on the positive, keep the peace, and enjoy the little moments, you give your loved one a meaningful, enriching quality of life.

## WHAT TO ASK THE DOCTOR

As always, write your questions in your notebook in advance, along with a list of current medications and dosages and information about any changes in health and behavior. Some things to discuss:

- How much should they eat, and what if they'll only eat certain foods like ice cream or toast with peanut butter? If their diet is very limited, how will that impact them?
- How much water should they be drinking?
- Is there medication that should be stopped or added?
- How will I know if they are in pain or have another illness?
- Do you have any suggestions for keeping them comfortable and preventing bedsores, infections, or illness?

# Self-Care

As your loved one declines, you may have noticed that you find yourself with more free time. They may be sleeping more often, and their days of running away or causing scenes in a restaurant may be behind them. However, the emotional baggage that comes with the late stage of Alzheimer's can be all-consuming and exhausting. It's still extra important to take care of yourself. When you've been gradually letting go, watching your loved change over time, it can result in feeling sad and generally worn out. Let's talk about how you can counter these effects when you:

- Focus on the positive
- Ask for and accept help
- Exercise thoughts and deeds of self-kindness

## FOCUS ON THE POSITIVE

Have you heard the line, "You can choose to have a good day or a bad day"? When you make a decision to focus on the positive, you tell your head and your heart that everything will be all right. It may not be perfect, and there may be tension and strife swirling nearby, but don't dwell on it—turn your energy toward the positive. A positive attitude will help you rise above the stress from external forces. Positive thinking is very powerful, and your mind, body, and health will thank you for it. It can lower your blood pressure, ease the impact of stress on your body, and provide you with great resilience when you need it most.

## ASK FOR AND ACCEPT HELP

Asking for help can be hard. As the disease has progressed, the level of care has increased. You may have already asked for help in some areas. When it comes to providing care for your loved one, no one does it better than you. When you ask for help, be prepared to accept it, even if the task may not be done the same way that you would do it. Take a moment and appreciate the effort—that someone else is taking the time to be with your loved one, even if it looks a little different. Accepting help takes tremendous strength and humility. Asking for help shows how brave you've become as a caregiver. Maybe you're in a scheduling pinch, or maybe you're totally exhausted, overwhelmed, and finally ready to accept some assistance. Regardless of the reason, try to accept the help, knowing that you'll be a healthier caregiver for it.

## EXERCISE THOUGHTS AND DEEDS OF SELF-KINDNESS

Being with your loved one as they enter the severe stage of the disease can take a toll on your emotional and physical health. It's been a long journey, and being gentle on yourself is more important now than ever before. You've been letting go, and with that comes all of the emotions that impact your health and wellness. Be kind and gentle with yourself, and get off your own back. Cut yourself some slack—you've done amazing work on this journey. No one is perfect, and your overall commitment has had a profound impact on your loved one. Now, give to yourself just as generously as you give to your loved one. You've provided care that is enveloped in love, tenderness, and kindness. Now, apply those exceptional attributes to yourself through thoughts and deeds of self-kindness.

### JUST ONE THING

You're focusing on the positive, letting go, and accepting help—or at least you're trying. These habits may take a little time to develop. Think about something that you can do right now for yourself. Think about one tiny thing that you can let go of. If your sibling is being a pain and not helping out, let it go. Then, treat yourself to something special as a reward. Go for a long walk, meet your friend for lunch, or go see a movie. If you can't get out, have a mini staycation—abandon the routine and stay in your pajamas all day. Take a bubble bath. Whatever you do for yourself today, do it without regrets—simply appreciate the moment—you deserve it.

> " The secret of health for both mind and body is not to mourn for the past, worry about the future, or anticipate troubles, but to live in the present moment wisely and earnestly."
> —BUKKYŌ DENDŌ KYŌKAI

# CHAPTER ELEVEN

# Nonverbal Communication

## NICK'S STORY

Tabby was called to become involved in the care of her father when he had already begun the severe stage of Alzheimer's disease. Tabby and her father were estranged for over 15 years. Nick had been a very angry man and wasn't active in Tabby's life. In fact, her mother left Nick when Tabby was just 7 years old, taking Tabby with her. The memories of her father were not good; all she could remember was him yelling all of the time. She had seen him a few times as she grew up, and then at her high school and college graduations, he gave her a $100 bill and said it was nice to see her. As time passed, her memories of him yelling started to fade as she moved on with her life.

Now, many years later, Tabby was called to see her father, who was living permanently in a nursing home. The big, loud man she remembered was now old and frail with gray hair and an ashen skin tone. When Tabby walked into the room, she said, "Hey, Dad." Nick looked up and gave a small smile; there was a moment of recognition in his eyes. Tabby wept and was instantly thankful that she had decided to come and see him.

## What to Expect

The damage to the brain from Alzheimer's disease will cause your loved one to become fully dependent on others for care. This care will include helping with activities of daily living, such as grooming, going to the bathroom, bathing, wiping, and cleaning themselves. "Full care" is the level of care provided in nursing homes and long-term care facilities. Generally, for full care to be provided, it takes a team to meet all the needs of your loved one, and this is a 24/7 responsibility. Your loved one will have increased difficulty with mobility, and eventually they will be unable to walk.

Communication will look very different as you accompany your loved one on this part of the journey. In the severe stage of the disease, your loved one will eventually lose the ability to speak. Related to this particular physical change in your loved one, you'll need to keep an eye on their ability to chew and swallow food and fluids. Choking can become a serious problem as the disease progresses into the severe stage.

As the level of care increases, your role will shift. The type of care needed will be based on keeping your loved one comfortable and staying connected to them. Helpful caregiving principles at this stage include:

- Closeness beyond words
- The importance of touch
- Eyes closed, ears and heart open
- New and quieter ways of being together

At this stage, you'll recognize that the busyness of caregiving that has been the norm for a long time starts to slow down. Yes, they'll need care around the clock, but the pace will change considerably. Whether your loved one is still at home or has transitioned to a skilled care facility, the type of care will be different.

## CLOSENESS BEYOND WORDS

This part of caregiving requires an entirely new approach that may feel very strange to you. For the past several years, you've been so busy helping, caring, coordinating, and taking care of just about everything. Now, even though your loved one needs full care, the approach needs to be slower, calmer, and more observant. When your loved one can no longer communicate in the way that they're used to, you'll want to find new ways to connect and respond to other signs and methods of communication. You know your loved one, probably better than anyone else. Pay attention to them, watch for physical responses or gestures—a slight smile or a turn of their hand with their palm facing up. When their eyes are open, look for that sparkle. When you see it, engage them gently; smile to offer comfort, support, and appreciation for them. When you're helping dress them, have them wear their favorite comfy clothes to preserve their dignity and identity.

The closeness to your loved one will move beyond words, because you know what will make them happy and content. This commitment has given you the unique opportunity to help provide the most intimate care for your loved one, and as your closeness transcends the spoken word, your actions will speak much louder than words ever could.

## THE IMPORTANCE OF TOUCH

One of the most profound acts of kindness that you can give is the gift of touch. Gently holding their hand as you talk to your loved one will help keep you both connected. Ever so slightly patting their hand, arm, or shoulder will help your loved one know that you care and are close by. Another role that you may take on is that of a teacher to others. Tell other family members or visitors that gently holding their hand and softly talking to them is a good thing. This allows other family members to stay connected, too. For those who are not accustomed to seeing your loved one in the severe stage of the disease, instruct and encourage them in their approach; this can alleviate tension and uncomfortable feelings. Your loved one needs the closeness of touch more than ever. Some people who visit may be afraid that they'll hurt your loved one if they touch them. Be patient with your explanations to those who may be afraid or not understand the disease.

## EYES CLOSED, EARS AND HEART OPEN

Your loved one now experiences the world through their senses. The sensations of touch, smell, sight, sound, and taste all help keep your loved one comfortable and calm in the severe stage of the disease. If their eyes are closed, research tells us they can still sense what is happening in the space around them. If people are arguing, their heart rate may increase and they may get agitated, so it's very important to keep their world free of stress and strife. Keep discussions about sensitive topics out of the room, away from them. Their body may be trapped, but their heart is open—don't underestimate what they can feel as a result of the environment.

## NEW AND QUIETER WAYS OF BEING TOGETHER

As the disease progresses and your responsibilities shift once again, you'll discover new, creative ways to be together. These will be calmer and quieter moments for you to share. For your loved one, maintaining their dignity must be the primary focus of all interactions. Slowing down and being open to adjusting your routine will help preserve their quality of life. Quality of life looks very different now. You've watched the progression of the disease change your loved one. You probably have changed as well. In the severe stage, this is the time to embrace yet another new norm. Be open to learning new ways to cope. Think about the laughter, the stories, and the moments you've shared with your loved one. Revisit the fond and comforting memories that you both have shared, both in your head and aloud so your loved one can hear. It's been a long journey, and now is the time to find the joy together in a quieter, softer way.

### INSIDE ALZHEIMER'S

As the disease progresses into the severe stage, the brain can no longer tell the body what to do in many functions. The functional impairment is so devastating that care is needed around the clock. The loved one can no longer be left alone. The interesting phenomenon about Alzheimer's disease is that your loved one may still react to music, or to their favorite pet. Their emotional memory can still be partially intact, and indeed, the brain may still respond to sensory stimulation, even in the severe stage of Alzheimer's disease. When they are exposed to familiar and pleasant sounds, such as a baby laughing or a cat purring, this can be very soothing.

## What to Say

Although your loved one may no longer have the ability to respond verbally to what is being said, you can still speak to them in a loving and reassuring tone.

*"Dad, I'm going to run to the pharmacy. The nurse will be here while I'm out. I'll be back in a little while." (If the nurse is a home*

*health aide or hired worker, you may not need to explain this; just keep it simple and concise.)*

*"Honey, you may have had an accident, let me help you change your clothes so you'll be comfortable. I want you to be warm, clean, and dry." (Then put on some music while you're changing their clothes.)*

*"Dad, I'm going to raise the bed up so you can have a sip of water. Maybe we'll have some ice cream later."*

*"Dad, your hands are so warm today. Remember the time we went sleigh riding and we froze our noses off? That was so much fun."*

And sometimes, the most powerful moments are silent ones.

## What to Do

Your loved one may not call you by your name anymore. Instead, appreciate that you can make them smile and that you see that spark in their eyes even for a moment. You can play and sing or hum along to their favorite song, knowing in your heart that it brings immense pleasure to them. You may not be able to carry a tune, but you can still sing or hum it anyway, then laugh a little at yourself and hope that no one is recording you.

Sharing the softer joys of life with your loved one will keep you connected. Put some flowers or a few fresh cut evergreen branches in a vase—that will bring a pleasant, natural fragrance to the room. Open the curtains and let the sun shine in.

If possible, bring your loved one outside to enjoy the fresh air, or open the window for them. Make the room comfortable for your loved one—this is important when they can't speak or do things for themselves. Letting sunlight in is a good practice. You know your loved one's preferences; keep it as consistent as possible to provide steady, reliable comfort and care.

Here are some other ways you can provide comfort:

- Music can be one of the most comforting sensations for your loved one in the severe stage of the disease. Put some on.
- Rub their favorite scented lotion on their hands.
- Wash and comb their hair if this will comfort them.

- Hold hands—this can be comforting for both of you.
- Help them pet their favorite animal—for some, the best comfort has fur and four legs.

## WHAT TO ASK THE DOCTOR

It may become very difficult to physically get your loved one to the appointment. Keeping them comfortable is the primary goal in the end stage. The final stages may not require seeing the doctor. You may be able to call the doctor and work with them to coordinate care needs over the phone. However, if you do go, bring your notebook with your questions written down in advance, along with a list of medications and dosages. Tell the doctor about changes in behaviors and the possible triggers.

Other questions might include:

- Can any medications be stopped at this point?
- How long do you think my loved one has to live?
- Should they be moved?
- How do I know I'm meeting their needs adequately?
- Do we need to come back or schedule another appointment?
- What if they have problems swallowing?
- Can I call if I have questions?

# Self-Care

You're learning new ways to communicate with your loved one and working to make them feel loved and comfortable. You're engaging their senses and keeping them connected with their environment and the people who are close by. Think about engaging your own senses to help relieve the strain of caregiving. What's *your* favorite lotion or scent? Maybe it's lavender, or lemon, or roses. Perhaps it's cinnamon or vanilla, or a combination of both that you love so much. Maybe it's spearmint or cool peppermint that makes you happy.

Taking care of yourself may now look different than it once did. Take a moment to reflect and revisit a time when you experienced something that made you very happy and content. Maybe you went to a concert or a play, or saw one of your favorite bands. Can you access the music? Listen to it—you'll feel better. Your self-care is still very important; it's been a long journey.

Equally important for you is not to isolate yourself. Stay connected to others to help keep you grounded and feeling supported on this difficult journey. You may realize that weeks or months have passed by, and you've been so dedicated to being a caregiver that you haven't seen your best friend or spent time with your partner. Part of self-care is surrounding yourself with love and support. Perhaps you can only face one person right now and not a group of people. That's perfectly fine. Carve out an hour or more, if possible, to get out, take a break, cry, laugh, do something silly, stand in the rain, catch snowflakes on your tongue, stick your toes in the sand, or walk barefoot on the grass. Then, take some deep breaths and tell yourself that you are very special, and you've got this.

## JUST ONE THING

As you engage your senses and those of your loved one, do one thing for yourself today. Take a moment to enjoy all for yourself. Retreat within. Close your eyes and meditate, or just breathe deeply for 10 minutes. Put on your headphones or earbuds and immerse yourself in your favorite song. You have more than earned the time to do just one thing for yourself today, or perhaps two ...

 I've learned that people will forget what you said, people will forget what you did, but people will never forget how you made them feel." —MAYA ANGELOU

# CHAPTER TWELVE

# Hospice

## ISAIAH'S STORY

When Isaiah and Mona met in their 50s, she became the love of his life. They have been together for over 21 years, never formally married, but deeply committed to each other. After 16 years together, Mona started to notice that Isaiah was becoming increasingly forgetful and misplacing important items. Isaiah was diagnosed with Alzheimer's disease, and it has taken just seven years to progress. Isaiah is at the end of his life, and Mona wants to be sure he is comfortable and well cared for. As the progression of the disease was somewhat rapid, Mona is working to make sure all of Isaiah's affairs are in order as she cares for him at the end of his life.

## What to Expect

How do you know when it is time to make the decision about placing your loved one in hospice care? Hospice care is the specialized care given to the terminally ill. It can be provided in the home or in a hospice facility. In the final stages of Alzheimer's disease, your loved one is very vulnerable to infections, especially pneumonia. If they've become incontinent, which is likely, it'll be important to make sure your loved one is clean and dry to protect the skin and reduce the risk of skin tears, bruising, and skin breakdown. Using proper absorbent and protective products is an important part of the care plan. It may be time to bring in more people to help with this type of specialized personal care. Very often, this is when hospice is called in. This decision can be difficult, but it may help you provide the best care for your loved one.

Some factors you'll want to consider:

- Talking to family members
- Making the decision
- Comfort care
- At home or out of home

## TALKING TO FAMILY MEMBERS

When you consult family members about bringing in hospice services, you are clearly indicating that this is the end of your loved one's life. It's imperative to know who's on your team. When you're talking to family about end-of-life care, this emotional subject can escalate very rapidly. At first, you'll want to enlist only those people who will really help you work this out. When you know your best allies, you'll want their support and assistance when talking about end of life.

If you have a complicated family situation, as many people do, first, gather information about the services and support that will best meet the needs of your loved one. Be prepared to explain what you've learned when you reach out to other members of the family, especially those who may be difficult. You may find that some relatives will come out of the woodwork when they learn that your loved one is in the final stage of their life. Surround yourself with a few people who will have your back when the time comes to talk to family members.

## MAKING THE DECISION

Making the decision to choose hospice can be incredibly difficult; conversely, you may find that the decision feels like the right thing to do. What you should know is that hospice provides an interdisciplinary team of experts who will help care for your loved one with dignity and respect. Assistance is provided for the caregiver as well, through counseling services and spiritual support.

Hospice will help you recognize the signs of dying. Hospice services also include bringing in durable medical equipment that may be needed to keep your loved one comfortable, such as a hospital bed. Nurses are available to make medication adjustments and care plans as your loved one's needs change. Personal care aides can help with bathing, grooming, and other personal care. Hospice social workers can help organize other resources that will benefit your loved one. There is also an opportunity for your loved one to make spiritual connections if they so choose, with the help of a spiritual advisor. When a family decides to have hospice involved, it doesn't mean that they give up all control or all hope. The focus of hospice is to provide comprehensive care that allows your loved one to live their final days comfortably and calmly with effective symptom management.

## AT HOME OR OUT OF THE HOME

Providing end-of-life care requires specific skills that must be balanced with sensitivity and a commitment to ensuring that your loved one's quality of life is preserved. When you've been the primary caregiver for many years, the care needed at this stage may be upsetting to provide. If the decision is made to keep your loved one at home at the end of their life, it's important to have a plan and be prepared if a crisis occurs or when the time comes for your loved one to pass away. Planning to keep your loved one at home may be the ideal goal. If your loved one has other co-occurring medical conditions that make providing care at home complicated, a team of people may be required to provide the appropriate level of care for your loved one. That would be the time to move your loved one to a hospice home or a long-term care facility that provides hospice services. Some hospitals have a few hospice beds on-site. Whether the decision is made to keep your loved one at home or move them to a location with a higher level of care, remember that keeping your loved one comfortable, calm, and well cared for is the goal.

## INSIDE ALZHEIMER'S

At the end stage of Alzheimer's disease, the brain is very severely damaged, and the body is no longer able to complete the most basic functions. The brain cannot send the necessary messages that provide direction for most parts of the body. As an example, when your loved one tries to eat, the tongue may no longer "know how" to accept food, and choking becomes a serious problem. The body cannot function, as a result of the damage to the brain. Music may be soothing, and quiet talking can bring comfort. Medically, your loved one is quite frail and susceptible to infections and injuries. Stepping into their shoes means being confined to bed and requiring full care for all needs. In the last stage of Alzheimer's disease, your loved one will require special care to ensure that respect, dignity, and physical comfort are provided until the end of their life.

## What to Say

Your words should focus on providing comfort in a peaceful environment for your loved one.

> *"Mom, we love you so much. The doctor recommended that hospice come in to help us take care of you."*

> *"Mom, the nurse and social worker from hospice will help us make a plan to keep you as comfortable as possible."*

For family conversations:

> *"Mom has been suffering from Alzheimer's disease for many years. It's time to let her go, and hospice will help us keep her comfortable."*

> *"Mom's doctor recommended hospice to help give her the level of care that she needs right now."*

> *"We can't keep Mom at home anymore—the ambulance has been here four times in the past three weeks. We can't take care of her anymore.*

*It's too hard for Mom to go to the emergency room every time something happens. It's the hardest decision we've ever had to make."*

*"I promised Mom that I would keep her home and never place her in a nursing home. She keeps getting infections, and I can't keep her comfortable anymore. The round-the-clock care is becoming too much, and I can't see her suffer anymore. Mom needs a team of professionals to help keep her comfortable. I'm devastated, but it's the right thing to do for her."*

## What to Do

What you can do is keep your loved one comfortable. It's been a long journey, and you've done so much. Keep the stress and tension away from your loved one. Speak to the hospice staff as often as needed; they are available 24/7 and will provide support for you as well as your loved one. Either keep family members informed, or designate someone for them to call besides you. Look at who is on your team, and delegate some tasks to help free up your time so you can spend it with your loved one as they come to the end of their life. Keep their pet close by, or items that you know will bring comfort to them. Pay attention to communication that is unspoken; this can be the most powerful method for staying connected to your loved one. Gentle touches, music, and soft talks about fond memories will bring comfort to all who are present.

### WHAT TO ASK THE DOCTOR

If your loved one is still seeing a doctor, bring your notebook with your questions, list of medications, and dosages. Talk to the doctor about any medical changes or changes in behavior.

Some things you might ask:
- Is it time for hospice?
- Are there other options besides hospice?
- How will we know when it's time to let them go?
- How will we know when they are about to pass away?
- Is there anything else I could be doing for them at this stage?

# Self-Care

At the end of the severe stage of Alzheimer's disease, finding peace with the situation can be one of the greatest gifts that you give yourself. When you make huge decisions that impact the life and care of your loved one, be gentle with yourself. Please know that you've done everything you could, to the best of your ability. Calling hospice can be really difficult, so get some support with this. Talk it out with a trusted friend. You've been letting go, a little at a time; this is another level of letting go. Treat yourself with care by avoiding negativity in others. If you must interact with difficult family members, keep this to a minimum and try really hard not to engage in battles—save and preserve your precious energy. Limit unnecessary conversations and interactions with toxic people. You are very special and do not deserve to be judged or criticized. It's been a long journey, and you've done well. Accept the fact that your caregiving has made all the difference. Your dedication and commitment have improved the quality of life for your loved one. Your self-care must continue to be a priority at this time, when the emotional drain on you is particularly intense.

### JUST ONE THING

You've been making difficult decisions, so today, think about making an easier decision: to do something nice for yourself. Pamper yourself; maybe get some extra sleep or take a nap. Take a break from the responsibilities and call your best friend, talk awhile, and share a belly laugh. Lighten up, and take some time just for yourself.

66 Laughter opens the lungs, opening the lungs ventilates the spirit." –UNKNOWN

# CHAPTER THIRTEEN

# Honoring Final Wishes

## RUTH'S STORY

Ruth was 81 and lived a good life. She raised four children and was a beloved teacher who worked with third- and fourth-grade students. She had a reputation of being firm but fair, and she loved children. Ruth was diagnosed with Alzheimer's disease when she was 70 years old. Her children were able to take care of her at home until the last six months of her life, when she was moved to a nursing home because the family could no longer manage her multiple medical conditions. It required a team to actively provide the 24/7 care needed to keep her comfortable. The family chose a facility near them, and they visited her almost every day. Ruth received good care; it wasn't perfect, but the staff did their best to provide a loving environment. Ruth could no longer walk, so she wasn't placed in the secure, locked unit where most people with Alzheimer's lived to prevent people from wandering out. Ruth was not a wandering risk. She had a semi-private room and lived there until she passed away.

## What to Expect

This part of the caregiving journey can involve emotional moments, difficult decisions, and family issues. However, the most important tasks are to respect and honor your loved one's final wishes. When you talk to your loved one about their final wishes, this can be emotional and uncomfortable, but it's necessary, as it will help you and the family plan and complete advanced directives. Ideally, you'll have already had these conversations before the end stage. By learning what your loved one wants at the end of their life, you won't have to guess and hope that you get it right. If there are resources such as a house, money, or a car, getting finances in order will be essential. Religious and cultural considerations should be discussed to ensure that traditions are honored and respected. Knowing your loved one's wishes will help minimize family disagreements and keep the peace.

In this chapter, we'll touch on issues including:

- Advanced directives
- Religious and cultural expectations
- Brain donation
- Funeral plans

## ADVANCED DIRECTIVES

Advanced directives are the legal documents that must be completed to memorialize your loved one's preferences at the end of their life. Ideally, these documents should be completed before your loved one enters the severe stage of Alzheimer's disease. The documents are called living will, power of attorney (POA), and health care proxy. For most families, these documents are completed when their loved ones are going through the middle stage of the disease (see Planning Ahead, page 59). The POA, which allows a designated person to manage the finances on behalf of your loved one when they are still living, becomes void immediately upon the passing of your loved one.

Advanced directives can vary by state, and you should enlist the help of an elder law attorney, if possible. Many county offices for aging have free legal clinics for seniors that may be available for you to access. Having these documents completed will help you honor your loved one's wishes.

## RELIGIOUS AND CULTURAL EXPECTATIONS

As the primary caregiver, you're probably well aware of the religious and cultural traditions that are expected to be carried out at the end of your loved one's life. Sometimes, people choose to reconnect with their faith community, seeking out spiritual comfort as they approach the end of life. You will need to act on behalf of your loved one when they can no longer express their wishes. You will be their advocate by providing the voice needed to ensure that their wishes are carried out properly.

## BRAIN DONATION

When the time comes and your loved one passes away, you might consider donating their brain for research purposes. If this is your loved one's wishes, your doctor will help you connect to an appropriate hospital. This is a difficult and tremendously sad decision to make for the family. However, if this is something you're willing to consider, recognize that brain donations assist in a type of research that can contribute to finding a cure and understanding how and why the disease progresses in the brain. When you're stressed and grieving, this decision can be incredibly overwhelming. Try not to get stressed about this decision—it sounds silly to say, but keep this in perspective. Most families know what their loved one would say—either yes, I'm okay with that, or absolutely not, no way do I want my brain donated for research. It's an option, but do not let this be the source of stress or family strife.

## FUNERAL PLANS

You may know how your loved one would like to be remembered. Planning the funeral or memorial service can be a rewarding opportunity to pay your final respects in a loving and personal way. You probably know what your loved one would want, and honoring those wishes is a very special gift that you can give. Turn to the people on your team to help you get through this very difficult time and emotional process.

At the very end of Alzheimer's disease, the brain is no longer able to provide the life-sustaining functions that are needed to survive. Your loved one will lose the ability to make facial expressions and communicate their needs. This can be very challenging for you to experience. There is no cure for Alzheimer's disease, and this will be the cause of their death, unless another medical situation causes fatal complications. As the end approaches, your loved one will need gentle comfort, good quality care, and your ever-present love and support.

# What to Say

Thinking about what to say to your loved one at the end of their life can be scary and overwhelming. On the other hand, you may be quite comfortable talking to your loved one, even at the end of their life. This is a very special and deeply emotional time to share. Consider the following statements:

> *"Dad, we want you to be comfortable. Relax and take it easy. We love you, and everything will be all right."*

> *"Dad, I pulled out the legal documents that we put together last year. I want to make sure your wishes are fulfilled."*

For family conversations:

> *"Dad said that he wanted to stay at home as long as possible, unless we couldn't take care of him anymore. We need to think about either bringing in more help to provide round-the-clock care or moving him. I promised I would never put him in a nursing home, but I can't take care of his medical needs anymore."*

*"It may be time to start thinking about making plans to pay our final respects to Dad. The doctor thinks he may be passing soon. Can you please call the family from out of town and tell them to come?"*

*"We all know what Dad wanted. Let's do our best to respect his wishes. This is so hard—more difficult than I ever expected."*

*"Dad is 85. He lived a good life, but it doesn't make this any easier."*

## What to Do

In the end stage of Alzheimer's disease, your loved one continues to experience their environment through their senses. Playing their favorite music or reading a few pages from their favorite book can still provide comfort. Rub a small amount of body-temperature lotion on their skin—this can feel very soothing, especially with the touch of your hands. The closeness that you share is indeed very special at this time. Think about ways that you can share treasured moments at the end of their life.

Be sure to have all the legal documents nearby. The advanced directives will guide the decisions that you'll be making at the end of your loved one's life. This can be a very demanding time for you, so it is essential to have a plan when your loved one needs more care or you need to move them. Being bounced from the hospital to a facility, then back home will cause high levels of stress and expose your loved one to potential infection and injury, as well as increased confusion and overall distress. It's important to keep an eye on your loved one to look for signs of distress and discomfort. If you notice changes in facial expression, swelling, or other physical signs that they might be in distress, call the doctor immediately. In the end stage of the disease, comfort and quality of life must be the priority. This is also a very special time for you to sit quietly with your loved one and cherish the final moments that you'll physically spend together.

## WHAT TO ASK THE DOCTOR

By now, your loved one will most likely not be seeing a doctor in person. Keep the doctor's phone number next to the phone or posted in a centrally located place.

You can call the doctor with the following questions:

- What medication should be stopped by this stage?
- What should I look for, or how will I know when my loved one is close to the end of their life?
- Is there anything else I can be doing to make sure they are comfortable? How can I ease any suffering?
- If my loved one passes away at home, must they still be transported to the hospital?
- Will you help us make a hospice plan that will provide the best type of care and at the appropriate place?

# Self-Care

For you, as the caregiver, this has been a long and difficult journey, but not without rewards. You've cared for your loved one and maintained their dignity and quality of life. That is the most precious gift you can ever give. You may not think so, but now is a good time to give yourself a break, even as your loved one is nearing the end of their life. Take a moment to laugh a little, cry a little, reminisce, and recognize that you've done an amazing job of caring for your loved one day after day. You've learned so much, accomplished a great deal, and been a true advocate for your special loved one. You may have surprised yourself with your strength and resolve. Even still, you must take some time to rest and to eat some healthy, nourishing food. Nourish your spirit and feed your soul to help strengthen yourself for this final part of the journey. This will be an emotionally and mentally draining time for you. You may see your loved one suffer at the end of life, and you'll want to be strong and reassuring for them.

Surround yourself with people who will love and support you! Taking care of your mind, body, and spirit is more important than ever. Paying attention to self-care will help keep you balanced to a certain degree. Make choices that are healthier for you, and resist any urge to turn to unhealthy habits to help cope with this devastating situation. If you do overdo something, immediately forgive yourself and get back on track the next day. Do not allow yourself to live with regret or self-doubt. You have been a devoted and thoughtful caregiver. No one's perfect, and when you're exhausted and worn out, you're particularly vulnerable to unhealthy coping mechanisms. Make a conscious effort to focus on your self-care in a positive and loving way.

Save your precious energy for the important tasks that need to be completed. Don't get caught up in family drama. Your self-care will help you manage your emotions and maintain balance during this time.

## JUST ONE THING

You have done some remarkable things, and your commitment has made a positive and profound impact on your loved one. Caregiving can pull at your emotions, especially toward the end of the long journey. Do one thing for yourself today. You are incredibly special and deserve some time to appreciate that. Go outside and breathe deep, rich, full breaths. Tip your face up to the sky and let the sun warm your face.

66 Some of us think holding on makes us strong, but sometimes it is letting go." –**HERMANN HESSE**

# Reflect and Look Ahead

You've completed the journey of being a caregiver to your loved one with Alzheimer's disease, and I don't need to tell you that it was no easy task. You may still be caring for your loved one and have finished this book now in order to understand some of what's to come. Or, maybe your loved one has passed, in which case I'm so sorry for your loss. As you well know, it's been a marathon, not a sprint, and you've done an extraordinary thing. Your time, energy, and love are the most precious gifts that you can share with another human being—and you have committed yourself to this noble cause in a most enduring way. Go ahead and shed tears for your loss, but hold your head up high for the courage and fortitude it has taken you to face the countless situations that you've encountered and met head-on. Hold dear the memories of time well spent, of challenges overcome, and of all the good times that you shared as you helped your loved one maintain a dignified and comfortable quality of life. That would not have happened without your love and commitment! You are so very special, and you can feel immensely proud of the difference that you've made in your loved one's life. Were there moments that you would have handled differently? Probably, and that's okay. Please place any regrets to rest, and find peace and comfort in the fact that you were doing your daily best in a prolonged and deeply challenging situation.

Turn your sights now to the future, being thankful for the life experience and feeling empowered with the knowledge that you are one tough, courageous, and resilient person, capable of accomplishing great things. You may never be the same again. Actually, you may find that you look at life a little differently. Things that bothered you in the past may be irrelevant now. You know who you can trust and depend on, and you are all the wiser as a result of this journey. You may discover that you'll be more inclined than ever to find appreciation in simple things. It's been quite a journey! You've grown, given, loved, and sacrificed your heart, and now it's time to appreciate all of the good work that you've done and the strong person you are today.

In all of it, remember to be good to yourself—you are, indeed, a hero!

> " If we celebrate the years behind us, they become stepping stones of strength and joy for the years ahead." —ANONYMOUS

# References

Alzheimer's Assocation. "Stages of Alzheimer's." Accessed February 11, 2019. www.alz.org/alzheimers-dementia/stages.

Alzheimer's Society. "What Are the 7 Stages of Alzheimer's Disease?" Accessed February 11, 2019. https://www.alzheimers.net /stages-of-alzheimers-disease.

Centers for Disease Control and Prevention. "What is Alzheimer's Disease?" Accessed February 11, 2019. https://www.cdc.gov/aging /aginginfo/alzheimers.htm.

Mayo Clinic. "Alzheimer's Stages: How the Disease Progresses." Accessed February 11, 2019. https://www.mayoclinic.org/diseases -conditions/alzheimers-disease/in-depth/alzheimers-stages /art-20048448.

National Hospice and Palliative Care Organization. "Hospice Care." Accessed February 11, 2019. https://www.nhpco.org/about /hospice-care.

Post, Stephen. "Why Deeply Forgetful People Matter: Hope, Ethics, and Individuals with Dementia." Dementia Training Australia. https://www.dta.com.au/wp-content/uploads/2017/10/DTA_Hope -and-Deeply-Forgetful-People-by-Professor-Stephen-Post.pdf.

# Resources

Caregiver support websites:

AARP.org/caregiving (AARP Resources for Caregivers and their Families)

ALZ.org/help-support/caregiving and ALZ.org/help-support /resources/helpline (Alzheimer's Association—the best place to go for accurate information about everything related to Alzheimer's disease, written by experts)

Alzheimers.org.uk (Alzheimer's Association, United Kingdom)

AMC.edu/patient/services/neurosciences/alzheimers_disease /index.cfm (Center of Excellence for Alzheimer's Disease at Albany Medical Center)

Caregiver.org (Family Caregiver Alliance)

www.Caregiver.va.gov (Veteran's Affairs Caregiver Support)

CaregiverAction.org (Caregiver Action Network)

Caregiving.org (National Alliance for Caregiving)

Facebook.com (Search for caregiver support groups in your area)

Health.harvard.edu/newsletters (Harvard Health Newsletter)

NADSA.org/learn-more/about-adult-day-services (National Adult Day Programs)

NIA.NIH.gov (National Institute for Aging)

NIH.gov (National Institute for Health)

ProjectLifesaver.org (Project Lifesaver)

SPHP.com/alzcare (Alzheimer's Caregiver Support Initiative for Northeastern New York)

WebMD.com (WebMD)

WHO.int (World Health Organization)

## HOTLINES

Alzheimer's Association (24/7) Helpline: 1-800-272-3900

## WEBSITES TO HELP WITH BENEFITS

DOL.gov/whd/fmla (Family and Medical Leave Act)

CMS.gov (Centers for Medicare & Medicaid Services)

Medicaid.gov/medicaid/ltss/self-directed/index.html (Medicaid)

## INSPIRATIONAL WEBSITES

Ted.com/talks (TED Talks)

## BOOKS

*Age in Place: A Guide to Modifying, Organizing and Decluttering Mom and Dad's Home,* by Lynda G. Shrager OTR, MSW, CAPS (Bull Publishing Company, 2018).

*The Caregiver's Toolbox: Checklists, Forms, Resources, Mobile Apps, and Straight Talk to Help You Provide Compassionate Care,* by Carolyn P. Hartley and Peter Wong (Taylor Trade Publishing, 2015).

*Coping with Your Difficult Older Parent: A Guide for Stressed-Out Children,* by Grace Lebow (William Morrow Paperbacks, 1999).

*Creating Moments of Joy Along the Alzheimer's Journey: A Guide for Families and Caregivers,* 5th ed., by Jolene Brackey (Purdue University Press, 2016).

*The Dementia Caregiver: A Guide to Caring for Someone with Alzheimer's Disease and Other Neurocognitive Disorders (Guides to Caregiving),* by Marc E. Agronin (Rowman & Littlefield Publishers, 2015).

*How to Care for Aging Parents, 3rd Edition: A One-Stop Resource for All Your Medical, Financial, Housing, and Emotional Issues,* 3rd ed., by Virginia Morris (Workman Publishing Company, 2014).

*Mike & Me: An Inspiring Guide for Couples Who Choose to Face Alzheimer's Together at Home,* by Rosalys Peel (Zadra Publishing, 2018).

*The Moral Challenge of Alzheimer Disease: Ethical Issues from Diagnosis to Dying,* 2nd ed., by Stephen G. Post (Johns Hopkins University Press, 2000).

*Passages in Caregiving: Turning Chaos into Confidence,* by Gail Sheehy (William Morrow, 2010).

*Somebody I Used to Know: A Memoir,* by Wendy Mitchell (Ballantine Books, 2018).

*Surviving Alzheimer's: Practical Tips and Soul-Saving Wisdom for Caregivers,* 2nd ed., by Paula Spencer Scott (Eva-Birch Media, 2018).

*The 36-Hour Day: A Family Guide to Caring for People Who Have Alzheimer Disease, Other Dementias, and Memory Loss,* by Nancy L. Mace and Peter V. Rabins (Johns Hopkins University Press, 2017).

*Thoughtful Dementia Care: Understanding the Dementia Experience,* by Jennifer Ghent-Fuller (CreateSpace Independent Publishing Platform, 2012).

*Understand Alzheimer's: A First-Time Caregiver's Plan to Understand & Prepare for Alzheimer's & Dementia* (Calistoga Press, 2013).

*When Reasoning No Longer Works: A Practical Guide for Caregivers Dealing with Dementia & Alzheimer's Care,* by Angel Smits (Parker Hayden Media, 2017).

# Index

Dignity, 81, 117, 136
Disinhibition, 92–93
Doctors
  finding the right, 58–59
  seeing multiple, 79–80
  what to ask, 26–27, 48, 60–61, 74, 85,
    95, 105, 118, 129, 138, 145, 154
Dressing, 80–81, 100
Drinking, 68
Driving, 42–43

E

Early detection, 16–18
Eating, 68, 102
Emotions, 37–38
End-of-life care, 141–145

F

Fall risks, 68–69
Family conflict, 114–115, 128–129, 142
Family Medical Leave Act (FMLA), 58
Final wishes, 149–150
Finances, 114–115
Franklin, Benjamin, 24
Full care, 133–134
Funeral planning, 151

G

Geriatricians, 59
Greenlee, Gina, 119
Grief, 124

H

Hallucinations, 91–92
Health care proxies (HCPs), 60–61, 150
Hesse, Hermann, 155
Hippocampus, 4
Hoarding, 41, 46
Home life
  long-term care, 116–117
  safety, 67–69, 72–73, 104–105
  simplifying the environment,
    46–47, 127
Hospice care, 141–145

Hospital beds, 128
Hypersexuality, 92–93

I

Incontinence, 127, 141
Instrumental activities of daily living
  (IADLs), 9, 15–16
Insurance, 63–64

J

Joy, finding, 125–126, 129

K

Kornfield, Jack, 30

L

Letting go, 124–125
Lifestyle habits, 7, 16
Living wills, 60, 150
Long-term care facilities, 117, 133–134

M

Medicaid, 64
Medical imaging, 61
Medicare, 64
Memory loss, 18–19, 36–37
Mercree, Amy Leigh, 75
Mild cognitive impairment (MCI),
  18–19, 54
Mild-moderate cognitive impairment,
  54–55
Music, 136–137

N

Neurologists, 58
Neurons, 3–4
Normal aging process, 18–22
Nursing homes, 133–134

P

Personal care, 80–81, 100–101, 117, 127,
  141–142
Personality changes, 41, 90
Planning ahead, 59–64

Positive thinking, 130
Power of attorney (POA), 61–62, 150
Present, being, 126, 129
Pressure ulcers, 127–128
Primary care providers (PCPs), 58
Public outbursts, 78–79

R

Religious traditions, 151
Retirement, 54–56
Routines, 46–47, 101

S

Safety, 43, 46, 68–69, 72–73, 104–105
Self-care, as a caregiver
　asking for help, 130–131
　building a support network, 64–65
　in the early stages, 29–30
　engaging the senses, 138–139
　finding peace, 146
　focus on the positive, 130
　importance of, 11–12, 106
　in the middle stages, 49–50

self-compassion, 65
self-kindness, 131
taking breaks, 74–75, 84–86, 96–97,
　107, 118–119, 154–155
Senior services, 58, 63–64, 104–105
Senses, engaging, 135, 138–139, 153
Singing, 80–81, 137
Sleep, 40
Socialization, 40
Suicidal thoughts, 39

T

Therapeutic fibbing, 100–101, 103–104
Tolle, Eckhart, 50
Touch, 135, 153

V

Veterans, 63

W

Wandering, 78, 102–103, 104
Working, 54–56

# About the Author

**Mary Moller, MSW, CAS,** has worked in the community for over 15 years, assisting families and caregivers as they try to balance the many demands placed upon them. Currently she works at the Center of Excellence for Alzheimer's Disease at Albany Medical Center. As a graduate of the Internship in Aging program at the School of Social Welfare at the University at Albany, where she earned her MSW, Mary has returned to the program as an adjunct professor and is pursuing her Ph.D. Mary has also earned a Certificate of Advanced Study in Health and Wellness.

In addition to her vast experience in aging and community-based social work, Mary has presented at many conferences on the topics of compassion fatigue and caregiver burnout, speaking to the importance of caring for the caregiver. Mary continues to make healthy aging and self-care a professional and personal priority.